A CANCER BATTLE PLAN

SIX STRATEGIES FOR BEATING CANCER FROM A RECOVERED "HOPELESS CASE"

ANNE E. FRÄHM WITH DAVID J. FRÄHM

JEREMY P. TARCHER/PUTNAM
a member of Penguin Putnam Inc.
New York

Most Tarcher/Putnam books are available at special quantity discounts for bulk purchases for sales promotions, premiums, fund-raising, and educational needs. Special books or book excerpts also can be created to fit specific needs. For details, write or telephone Putnam Special Markets, 200 Madison Avenue, New York, NY 10016; (212) 951-8891.

Jeremy P. Tarcher/Putnam
a member of Penguin Putnam Inc.
200 Madison Avenue
New York, NY 10016

First Jeremy P. Tarcher/Putnam Edition 1997
Originally published by Piñon Press, Colorado Springs, CO

Copyright © 1992 by Anne E. and David J. Frähm
Introduction copyright © 1997 by Anne E. and David J. Frähm
All rights reserved. This book, or parts thereof, may not be
reproduced in any form without permission.
Published simultaneously in Canada

Library of Congress Cataloging-in-Publication Data

Frähm, Anne E.
A cancer battle plan: six strategies for beating cancer from a
recovered "hopeless case" / by Anne E. Frähm
p. cm.
Includes bibliographical references.
ISBN 0-87477-893-X
1. Cancer—Popular works. 2. Cancer—Alternative
treatment. 3. Cancer—Nutritional aspects.
I. Frähm, David J.
RC263.F69   1998   97-25467   CIP
616.99′4—dc21

Printed in the United States of America
12 14 16 18 20 19 17 15 13 11

This book is printed on acid-free paper. ∞

Contents

To God, who saved me more than once

To my "cancer cousins," courageous in battle,
who have become free from cancer by graduating from life:

> *Harry Shisler*
> *John Wainscott*
> *Dick Tamulionis*
> *Ron Kaper*
> *Sue Montgomery*
> *Lynn Winkelhake*
> *Francis DiSimone*

Thank you to
Dr. David Headley,
Dr. George Juetersonke,
and my friend Yasmine Marca,
for their dedication to people's health

Acknowledgments

Although this book is written in my voice (Anne), let the truth be known. My husband, Dave, slaved over a hot computer for more than a year to bring about the feast that you now hold in your hands. My humble role as consultant and editor was puny in comparison. Without his gifted expertise, this book would have stayed in my mental file of good ideas. Thanks, honey.

I'd also like to thank my family and friends for coming to my side and strengthening my weak knees. They supported me in ways I can't begin to tell—except one. They prayed for me. Thanks for not giving up on me.

I wish I could take away the pain that my husband, children, and extended family members endured during my walk through the valley of the shadow of death. They suffered more than I. But I know that God has and is using all this for good in their lives. Thank you for hanging in there and taking care of me when I really needed it.

Introduction

When I first received the shocking news that I had cancer, my thirst for *hope* was akin to a person shipwrecked on a desert island without water. I had to have it! I just had to know that somebody out there had survived cancer as bad as mine. To live without hope was to curl up and die.

One of the first things I did when I was able to leave the hospital was go to the local library to acquaint myself with my enemy. I found 497 entries! Where to begin?

I started with my particular brand—breast cancer. As I pored over each book, it was easy for me to tell which ones were not worth my reading. Those that were filled with statistics that rang my death knell quickly found their way back to the shelves to gather more dust.

In others, I found bits and pieces of information that were more helpful. I learned that for every form of cancer, there was someone who had overcome it. That was just the hope I needed. From that point on I determined that I was going to fight. Although my prognosis was bleak, this was going to be the "Mother of All Battles"! I was going to use every resource available to beat this thing.

For a year and a half I read every book and underwent every conventional therapy—surgery, chemotherapy, radiation, and hormone therapy. Finally, presented as my last option, I underwent an autologous bone marrow transplant. When this, too, failed to send my cancer into remission, the medical world pronounced me "hopeless." Not ready to lie down and play dead, I turned elsewhere. Within five weeks after starting a strict program of detoxification and diet under the guidance of a nutritional counselor, my cancer had packed its bags.

This book is a distillation of all that I've learned about beating cancer in the face of little medical hope. I wish I'd found this book in the library that day when I'd gone looking for help and hope. I am confined, for legal reasons, to say that nothing in this book is to be taken as a claim to curative powers. Nonetheless, my hope is that information in this book will help you take responsible control of your health in such a way as to provide your body with what it needs to reverse cancer.

Introduction to the Second Edition

It's now been several years since these pages first made their way to bookstore shelves. Our Health*Quarters* Ministries organization, born in response to an ever-widening audience eager to learn more about using nutrition to achieve health, has been busy. Testimonies of healing resulting from practicing the principles outlined herein have poured in.

As for me, I'm doing great! I'm still working at ridding my body of toxins that have been stored for years in fat cells, but my health has never been better. And although my knowledge base concerning fighting cancer with "alternative" weapons has expanded, that base rests squarely on the guiding strategies you're about to discover.

As you work your way through this book, be sure to give HQM a call if we can be of any help or offer encouragement. We're here to serve you.

A War Story

The room was already darkened in the staff's hurried anticipation to get home to their loved ones. I was alone, except for a sole technician who busied herself in the next room with the sort of impatient sounds that told me she, too, had other places she wished to be.

Only minutes earlier a host of doctors and technicians had been scurrying about the room, sinking long needles into various places in my back, and passing my body in and out of a Cat-scan machine. "Does that hurt? Does that hurt?" they kept asking as they probed for whatever it was they were looking for along my spine. Finally, having located their target, a large syringe was employed, and a small amount of fluid was withdrawn.

As I lay there on the gurney waiting for the belated volunteer to return and wheel me ever so carefully back to my hospital room, two competing emotions washed back and forth across my mind. First a sense of relief. Finally, after so many months of agony and frustration, I would have real explanations of the incredible pain I was experiencing in my back. At last I would know for sure what I was dealing with. But then, what *was* it I was dealing with? The sense of fear was inescapable! Why had I not been getting better, but worse?

For most of the previous seven months, pain had been woven into the fabric of my daily existence. Shortly after Thanksgiving, I'd begun to notice the mysterious presence of a steady pain between my shoulder blades. The only remotely possible cause I could point to was a little "fender bender" just a few days earlier in which my car was rear-ended.

In January my husband and I decided to redecorate our kitchen. The night we completed the project, my left shoulder began to throb with excruciating pain. It felt as if I were being stabbed repeatedly with a large butcher knife. Subsequent weeks found me wearing a path in and out of our family doctor's office, complaining of increasing pain. My back hurt, my shoulder was killing me, and it was becoming increasingly difficult to walk.

His diagnosis? Bursitis of the shoulder, complicated by a kidney infection that was keeping fluid from properly draining from the muscles in my body. Inactivity was ordered, along with heavy doses of antibiotics. But as the weeks came and went, the suffering intensified. The painkillers I was forced to use for sleep were making mincemeat of my intestines. The number of sleepless nights mounted.

By mid-February, hospitalization was what the doctor ordered. X-rays showed "hot spots" on the bones of my shoulder, which were interpreted as the bursitis. Daily ice packs were given along with massive doses of IV-introduced antibiotics for the supposed ongoing kidney infection. After leaving the hospital, I kept my left arm in a sling for the entire month of March. Twice a week, for a month, I spent an hour at the hospital in the physical therapy unit getting cortisone treatments on my shoulder.

By April the pain was still increasing, dramatically!

What was happening to me? Why was I not getting better? Why wasn't this kidney infection clearing up? Here I was, only thirty-five years old and otherwise in good shape, yet crippled with debilitating pain. How long would I have to endure this torment before my body did a turnaround? Our family doctor continued to believe that as soon as the kidney infection was gone, the muscles in my back would return to normal function. In the meantime, rest and wait.

April and May were hellish! I began to spend most of my days and nights flat on my back in bed, just waiting for things to get better. Sometimes the pain in my back was so fierce that it was sheer agony to do the simplest things, like turn over—so I didn't. Sleep was nearly impossible. My husband was forced to make his bed on the floor of our bedroom, for even his slightest movements beside me in bed would trigger the muscles in my back, causing me to erupt in screams of agony. Just hearing our two children walk outside our bedroom door was enough to tighten my muscles into gripping spasms that made even breathing difficult.

That time was hard for my kids. They were not only worried about me, but angry that I demanded so much attention and could not act in motherly ways toward them. Both were in grade school and needed their mom to fill their emotional tanks with hugs and kisses. Instead they got daily doses of "Don't get too close!" "Don't touch the bed!" "Be careful, please!"

Fortunately, my husband's work was such that he could do it at home. He became both father and mother to our kids, and for me, full-time nurse. He cooked meals, washed clothes, kept house, and when I felt the call of nature, he assisted me to the bathroom. It usually took about fifteen minutes, with a lot of his help, to get from my bed to the bathroom door across the hall. The relief in my bladder was often overshadowed by the humiliation of needing Dave to help me lower my body onto the stool, then assist me to stand up when I was finished. As the days trudged by, even that became impossible.

Finally, one morning in late May, we'd had enough of this waiting around. We wanted to believe what our doctor was telling us, but things just weren't getting better. We didn't want him to think that we'd lost confidence in him, but we needed answers. That day we managed to get my tortured body out into the car and over to the emergency room of the local hospital. There, we thought, we'd be able to get another doctor's opinion on what was going on, perhaps even be admitted to the hospital for tests. Unfortunately, we received only more frustration for our efforts. After conferring with our family doctor over the phone about whether or not all this pain was really just in my head, the attending physician administered a shot of muscle relaxant and sent us away with a prescription for valium and advice that I do some slow walking to bring my muscles back to work again.

Thanks for nothing! We left there frustrated, knowing that we had not been helped. The next day we managed one last trip to our family doctor. This time we wanted new answers!

AND THE ANSWER IS . . .

The quietness that enveloped me, as I lay on the gurney in the Cat-scan room reviewing all that had led up to that moment, was suddenly broken as a young doctor thrust open the door and entered. He stood in the light that followed him from the hall, looking around in the semi-darkness until he spotted me.

Hurrying to my side, he said, "Hello, Mrs. Frähm? My name is Dr. S. I'm a surgeon. In fact," glancing at his watch, "I'm late for surgery. Mrs. Frähm, I hate to tell you this, but you have advanced breast cancer. You need a mastectomy, and I can fit you in at 5:30 p.m. tomorrow, okay?"

Upstairs in my hospital room, my husband was receiving the same news from a newly appointed oncologist. Stunned and emotionally overwhelmed, he managed to ask only one question—"How long does she have?"

"I'm not going to pull any punches. You need to know the truth," answered the oncologist. "Most people who have cancer as advanced as your wife's die within two years." (Only later did we learn from him that this had been highly optimistic.)

Finally, I was wheeled back to my room and placed in bed. With frightened eyes brimming with tears and hearts ready to explode, Dave and I clung to each other and wept. Can it be true? Is all of this really happening to us? Is my lifelong nightmare coming true?

We mourned my death.

A "FALSE NEGATIVE"

"False Negative" is the term used in the field of mammography when the results of a woman's mammogram show that the lump in her breast is not cancerous when in reality it is. Statistics show that ten to thirty out of every 100 women who have breast cancer receive false negatives.[1] These unfortunate women return home relieved with the news that they have nothing to worry about. Only later, as the cancer has a chance to grow, does it become apparent just how big their worries should have been.

Five months before the pain in my back became noticeable, I'd discovered, during a self-examination, a small lump in my left breast. My family history of breast cancer told me that these were not to be ignored. My grandmother had died of breast cancer. My mom, although never developing cancer, had experienced multiple recurrences of cysts in her breasts. Fearing the fate that had overtaken her mother, she'd undergone a double mastectomy when she was in her thirties. Needless to say, I called our family doctor immediately!

The mammogram I had at the local clinic spotted what were actually two tiny lumps and labeled them noncancerous, benign. An additional test, an ultrasound, also showed them as negative.

"Nope, no cancer here," was the doctor's verdict after the ultrasound test.

"How can you be sure?" I insisted.

"If a lump is cancerous, it shows up on the screen as a solid mass. These lumps, they're full of fluid. These are just cysts that you have nothing to worry about."

But only five months later aggressive breast cancer had begun to make itself known as the growing pain in my back. By the time I'd finally been admitted to the hospital for tests, the cancer—which had begun as two little lumps in my left breast—had spread throughout my body. Tumors were found covering my skull, my shoulder, my ribs, my pelvic bone, and up and down my spine—in addition to the huge tumor that had developed from those two little so-called "noncancerous" lumps in my breast. So aggressively had this cancer attacked my body, it had eaten a stress fracture right into my backbone. My back was actually broken!

The day after Dr. S. made his dramatic entrance into my life with the crushing news of breast cancer and my need for surgery, Dave and I insisted that we have time to talk with him before making this decision. He apologized for having been so abrupt, assuring us that he was interested only in what was best for me. In his mind I needed surgery, soon! His schedule was filling up fast. He didn't want to waste precious time with niceties.

As we interacted with him concerning my options, he said something that every woman needs to know. Something I wished somebody had told me nearly a year earlier when I'd discovered the lumps for the first time. "Don't trust the results of a mammogram or ultrasound," he said. "If you have a lump, *always* have it biopsied!"

SURGERY, RADIATION, CHEMOTHERAPY

I had the mastectomy. At precisely 5:30 that evening, my left breast was removed, along with a tumor beneath it the size of my entire breast. At the same time a hickman catheter, a fifteen-inch tube leading directly to my heart, was implanted in my chest, through which chemotherapy treatments were to be administered.

The next day, still groggy and hurting from surgery, I was hooked up to my first of many, many bags of chemicals designed to kill the cancer cells that had taken up residence in the rest of my body.

The picture wasn't a bright one. We were not happy campers. Life had fallen down around our knees, leaving us exposed and vulnerable. We felt helpless, hopeless, and hollow. Cancer had descended on us like a fog, leaving us groping our way toward the future. What do we do now? How long do I have? How shall we tell the kids? How should we live?

When I first received the news that I had cancer, my one burning question concerned whether or not there were other people with the disease as progressed as mine who had survived. If nobody had, I wasn't sure I even wanted to try.

On the other hand, I wasn't one who could simply throw in the towel and play the helpless victim. Such a thing would be contrary to my nature. I was a fighter. If there was any way for me to beat cancer, I was determined to find it.

After I was released from the hospital I went to the public library and immersed myself in books about cancer. Since there were 497 entries, I narrowed my research to my own disease—breast cancer. Many of the books were lofty commentaries filled with statistics that only a doctor could or would want to understand—books that coldly sang my funeral dirge. Back to the shelves they went to gather more dust. But in some books I found the stories of various individuals who had overcome every form of cancer there was. Some of these folks had made it back to life from their deathbed. With their encouragement and my own resolve to be an overcomer, I decided to fight my enemy with every ounce of my being.

For the next year and a half I aggressively subjected my body to all that the medical world had to offer in the battle against cancer. A couple of the larger tumors near my backbone were given two weeks of radiation. This, coupled with the chemotherapy, was more than my body could handle and landed me in the hospital with severe pneumonia. My body miraculously overcame that setback, and eventually I got back on the chemotherapy track. Actually, I tolerated chemo amazingly well. As promised, my hair fell out. I remained shiny bald for eighteen months. And the chemo made me very, very tired. But the positive effects it had against my cancer outweighed all the negatives.

For a time my cancer count went steadily downward toward remission. Things looked hopeful. I was grateful for the chemicals I was putting into my system to poison the cancer, looking on them as trusted friends. But about ten months into treatment, just as my oncologist had predicted, the chemo began to wane in its effectiveness. My cancer had grown resistant. A new blend of chemicals was tried. To this we added hormonal therapy. But each time counts were taken, it was obvious that the disease was gaining ground and I was beginning to lose the battle.

"There's a last resort you may want to consider," said my oncologist. "It's a bone marrow transplant. If you wish, I'll call a couple of hospitals where they do them and see if you're a good candidate."

BONE MARROW TRANSPLANT

A year and a month after my original diagnosis with cancer, and after three frustrating postponements, I was accepted into the bone marrow transplant program of a major Midwestern hospital. This was to be an "autologous" procedure. In other words, I was going to be my own donor. The treatment involved four steps. The first was to collect stem cells from my blood to be saved and reinjected into my body at a later point. Step two was to put me in an isolation room and bombard my cancer with massive doses of chemotherapy, many times stronger than my body could safely tolerate under other circumstances. The goal was to kill all the cancer in one powerful swoop. Step three was to reinject the reserved stem cells, hoping that they would take root and rebuild my bone marrow that had been destroyed along with the cancer in step two. Keeping me alive while my stem cells labored to multiply was the all-important goal of step four.

So, several hours a day for two weeks, I was hooked up to a machine that collected stem cells from my blood. Having completed that process, I was admitted into an isolation room to begin steps two through four. For the first seven days my system was saturated with chemotherapy. I was literally being killed on the inside. The chemo was getting after my cancer, but it was also destroying my good blood cells and immune system. Any sort of germ or infection that entered the room was a death threat.

My husband, kids, and mother had moved for the summer to the city where the hospital was located and were allowed to visit in the room, but they had to wear shoe coverings, gowns, rubber gloves, and face masks. I couldn't even have fresh flowers in the room, for fear that they might carry in some sort of bacteria.

At the beginning of my second week in isolation, the collection of stem cells that had been previously gathered was reintroduced to my body. The process of waiting for them to rebuild my now-destroyed bone marrow began. In all I spent fifty-two days in that room, much of which I don't remember. My husband has had to fill me in on nearly the entire month of July. The constant flow of drugs to help my body cope with the nauseating effects of chemo saturation and to guard it against infections left my brain numb. I don't even remember the emergency surgery mid-month when pneumonia had shut down my right lung and my kidneys had begun to fail. It simply didn't register in my head, when they wheeled me toward the operating room, that I was teetering on the edge between life and death.

My husband has reviewed with me the emotions of that night. The kids needed to be told that I was in very serious condition and might die shortly. He spoke to them gently, holding their hands in his, then putting his arms around them in a huddled mass of sobs and tears. It was very difficult for them all. He called friends back home, asking them to pray. My dad was notified and began making preparations to come. Together, Dave and our kids sat with my mom in the surgical waiting room, preparing themselves for the worst. Tears were shed, prayers offered, shoulders leaned on. A note Dave made in his pocket diary that night read "death predictable."

Hours passed as they waited to see what was to become of me that night. Finally, in the wee hours of the morning, the surgeon entered the waiting room and spoke to Dave. "The lung itself looks okay," he said. "We took a piece of it so we can see what's going on in there. Better go home and get some sleep now."

A betting man would have been wise not to put any money on my recovery. Most patients who die during this kind of a bone marrow transplant do so because of complications caused by pneumonia. It looked very much like I was about to join them.

I was being watched closely. Each morning a technician would wheel in a portable x-ray machine to take new pictures of my lungs. A twelve-inch tube had been inserted into my chest to drain the fluid from around my lung. Between that and the fact that the surgeon had pulled apart my ribs to get a good look, it hurt to even think about moving my arm, much less lie on my side.

The biopsy revealed nothing unusual, at least as far as making changes to the drugs I was being given. It never became apparent why the mix of antibiotics I'd been on from the start of the transplant procedure hadn't protected me from developing pneumonia. There was nothing to be done but to keep pumping me full of the same stuff and hope for the best.

Truly by the grace of God I began to get better. I attribute that to the prayers of friends and family who were appealing my case before the Creator. The hospital staff really didn't expect me to recover. I'll say more about the tremendous power of prayer later in this book. For now I want you to know that under all that is written in these pages is a very strong conviction that God has complete authority over each person's life.

As late July turned into early August, I began to gain back some of my strength. Things began to look hopeful. Perhaps I would survive this treatment after all. And I hoped all the cancer in me wouldn't. I hadn't eaten a thing for weeks, receiving my nourishment through an IV tube. Food was reintroduced to my daily routine. Gradually I began to be able to keep some of it down.

The coughing and vomiting, which had become a major part of my hourly existence during these weeks and months, had caused my eyes to go bloodshot. My left eye was so completely red that no white was visible. It was real sci-fi! It didn't hurt much, but visitors would cringe when they first saw me. I'd also developed a rash that covered me from head to toe with deep reds and brilliant purples. My skin had been burned from the inside out,

turning it eventually to a leathery brown. The outside
layer of my mouth and gastrointestinal tract blistered
and fell off. What a sight I must have been! Tubes running
in and out of my "bald headed, bloody eyed, covered with
splotches, decaying body." Yuck! Besides all these outer
manifestations, the massive amounts of chemotherapy
administered had taken a considerable toll internally.
Damage was sustained to all my vital organs.

One day, the time had come to do another bone
marrow biopsy, a painful procedure of inserting a long
needle deep into my hip bone to withdraw bone marrow.
Such a procedure had been performed on me before
I'd left home for the transplant. At that time cancer
cells had been found in my marrow. Checking it now
would tell whether the transplant had been a success—
whether going through this hell had been worth it.

The days that passed between the biopsy and getting
the results back did so slowly. Didn't the lab know how
important this news was to us? Finally the word came. They
had not been slow, but careful. There were some things in
the biopsy that they needed to take a closer look at.

"I'm so sorry," said the doctor, taking my hand, her
eyes welling up in tears. "There's still a lot of cancer in
your bone marrow." (A friend was later told by my doctors,
"Anne Frähm's just one of those unfortunate people for
whom the procedure didn't work. It was hopeless, really.")

That was a hard pill to swallow! The cancer was
still there. The procedure had not been as effective as
was hoped. It had killed a lot of the cancer cells, but
not all. What were left would be multiplying. Any more
chemotherapy was out of the question. According to the
doctors, it was only a matter of time before the cancer
would finally win the war.

It was hard to stay in that room for a couple more
weeks, doing nothing but waiting for my stem cells to graft
in enough to raise the blood-producing capacity of my bone

marrow. My white blood cell count teetered between zero and 100 for days. Normal is between 4,000 and 10,000. My count had to go up before I went into the "real world" filled with germs that only white cells could protect me against.

My mother heard that there was an experimental drug being tested on some of the patients in the ward that had the potential of stimulating growth of white blood cells. When I asked my doctor about it, his reply stunned me. "There is a limited amount of it available at this point for research," he said. "It's therefore being held in reserve for patients with a more favorable long-term prognosis than yours. I'm sorry."

It was as if he'd already put me in a coffin and was nailing it shut! Whatever wind was still in my sails might have left me at that point had I not had a strong belief that I was in God's hands and that, in any situation life presents us, there's always hope. A favorite verse from the Bible encouraged my confidence: "Do not fear, for I am with you; do not be dismayed, for I am your God. I will strengthen you and help you; I will uphold you with my righteous right hand."

Eventually the team of doctors on the ward decided that I was to be released. No, my white blood count had not yet reached a safe level to protect me against the germs of life, but there was no telling when it would. I might languish in the hospital for weeks. Besides that, they needed the room. A long list of others wanted to undergo the transplant procedure; others for whom it might be more successful. It was time for me to leave.

The morning of my emergence from the hospital, the doctors came in and gave me a little speech. It was a blend of cautions I needed to remember in order to protect myself against germs, mixed with cheery ideas about how good it would be for me to get back home and into living my life again. Basically what they told me was to go and live life to its fullest. I knew that behind their words was the unspoken prognosis that my time was short. "Eat, drink, and be merry," they were saying, "for soon you will die."

But as I've said, there's always hope! The doctors were giving me up as a "goner," but I wasn't ready to check out of life yet. I was in this fight to the finish! I wouldn't believe it was over until I'd met my Maker.

TURNING TO NUTRITION

Early in my cancer battle, I'd read about the link between cancer and diet. In fact, I'd visited a nutritionist in my hometown shortly after my chemo treatments began to see what she might have to offer. I warned her at the outset of our appointment that I wanted nothing negative to be said about chemo, maintaining my belief that having a positive attitude toward it made it more effective. What I wanted from her were ideas about nutritional practices that I might integrate into my overall program of treatment. When she began to talk about the potential need to cut back on dairy products and meat and a variety of other foods, I balked.

"Give up cheese?! I lived in Wisconsin for nine years. I've got cheese in my blood!" I complained.

I really can't remember what else we talked about that day. I guess my mind had closed itself off to whatever she thought was important to tell me. Giving up the kinds of foods that I liked so much seemed, at that point, too great a price to pay.

But now, back home from a less than totally successful program of treatment, which my oncologist had called my last resort, I had no other options. Cancer was growing back quickly in my system. My pelvic bones were beginning to hurt again, and my limp was returning. I'd traveled every path offered to me that intersected in some way with conventional cancer treatment. My résumé of therapies read like a medical textbook. I was now on the last page, with my life looking like it might be coming to a close. I gave the nutritional approach another shot.

I began a strict regimen of detoxification, diet, and sup-plements under the guidance of a nutritional counselor. Five weeks later tests done by my oncologist revealed no trace of cancer! He was flabbergasted!

"When you returned from the transplant with cancer still in your marrow," he said, "I honestly thought you were doomed!"

A VISION BORN
As my story circulates through the cancer-fighting grape-vine around the country, more and more people call to get the details of what worked for me. Several local doc-tors have given out my phone number in hopes that my experiences might give practical help and emotional encouragement to their patients with cancer. As a result, and because of a sense of personal calling to influence our world, my husband and I have begun our own nonprofit organization called HealthQuarters. Our hope is to fill the information, education, and encouragement needs of fellow "cancer cousins." With them I share the lessons I've learned about fighting cancer that fill the pages of this book, namely:

- *Know your enemy.*

- *Cut off enemy supply lines.*

- *Rebuild your natural defense system.*

- *Bring in reinforcements.*

- *Maintain morale.*

- *Carefully select your professional help.*

My hope is that you will find suggestions in these pages to help you win your own war on cancer. May God make it so.

II

Principle One—
Know Your Enemy

The headlines read, "Man Charged With Aiding Mom's Suicide." The story told the tragic details of a local man who'd given his mother a handgun so she could kill herself. The reason? Seems she'd just been diagnosed with cancer of the liver.

Cancer is the great "mystery" disease that we all crossed our fingers and hoped we'd never get, yet here we are. When we're first diagnosed, most of us don't know much about it or what causes it. We know only that many people seem to get it and die. In fact, current statistics reveal that one out of every three people in the United States will develop the disease. It's the number-two killer after heart disease, threatening to take over as number one.[1]

Being told that you have cancer is shocking enough, but when the diagnosis is followed by a doctor's prediction of your impending doom, absolute terror sets in. The physician of the woman in the newspaper article had informed her that she had but a month to live. Distraught and overwhelmed by the fear of an agonizing death, she took charge of her situation in the only way she knew how.

I, too, have experienced the emotional depths of being told that death was just around the corner. I've felt the frustration and heavy despair that comes from being told you're going to die and there's nothing much anyone can do about it. I've anguished over the realization that I may not get to see my children grow up, that my next Christmas may be my last, that my spouse may be left alone. Mine was widespread fourth-stage cancer, the worst. I've been through that emotional wringer.

But let me assure you that cancer need not be considered an automatic death sentence—no matter how bad you feel, no matter how unfavorable your prognosis. My success against the disease is not an isolated case. Many people have fought back to regain their health. Many people have conquered the disease in the face of overwhelming odds. You can take charge of your situation in ways that will help your body win its war. Cancer is a degenerative disease, and degenerative diseases can be reversed. *It's always too soon to give up!*

No one can, of course, give you an iron-clad guarantee that you'll be victorious. Life just doesn't work that way. Each body is unique; each situation different. The bulk of this book has to do with a detoxifying and nutrition-based rebuilding process that I undertook with success. Whether or not the same will work for you depends a great deal on the condition of your metabolic system, particularly your liver, and your body's eventual ability to utilize nutrients for self-healing (something the body is designed to do).

Unfortunately, at this time in medical history, many cancer patients don't turn to nutritional therapy until all so-called "conventional" options have been exhausted. Often the ravages of surgery, radiation, and chemotherapy have by that time so damaged their vital organs that their systems are simply unable to respond favorably to "self-healing" stimulation. But you just never know. I'm here as a testimony to the potential of nutritional therapy to help restore health even against the worst odds.

Obviously I can't provide you with a magic formula for beating cancer. What I can provide are the ingredients for a fighting chance. The first ingredient is *hope*—hope that the battle is not impossible. If it happened for me, as far gone with disease as I was, perhaps it will happen for you. The second ingredient is important *information* from cancer experts that you may be unaware of—information that has the potential to help you help your body win its battle. If you'll just add the *willingness* to do whatever it takes, it's possible you will get positive results, as I and many others have. It's worth your best shot, right?

In war, the better you know your adversary, the more likely you are to beat him. The same is true in battling cancer. The better your information about the disease, the greater your odds of overcoming it. With that in mind, let's take a look at what the experts are saying about cancer—what it is, what causes it, and what sort of strategy seems to make the most sense toward reversing it.

By the way, you need to know that during the autopsy it was discovered that the woman didn't have cancer after all, but an infection—pockets of pus on her liver. Seems she'd been misdiagnosed by her doctor. With proper medical attention she probably would have been fine. Sometimes, the greatest obstacle to regaining your health is misinformation about your problem. Read this chapter carefully.

WHAT IS CANCER?
The world of sickness, disease, and health problems can be divided into two lists: "acute" and "chronic."

Recently my son fell on a rain spout while playing kick-the-can with his buddies. The gouge in his side, requiring seven stitches at the local emergency room, was an acute health problem. It was the sudden onset of a previously nonexistent medical emergency. Broken bones are another example of acute health problems—as are cuts, scrapes, broken teeth, and bullet wounds. You get the idea. On the chronic list are health problems of a much different sort. Recurrent conditions like allergies are found here, as are degenerative diseases that develop in their host over an extended period of time without immediately noticeable symptoms. Various heart and circulatory diseases are on this list, as well as cancer. Cancer is a chronic degenerative condition in which normal cells have become chemically altered mutations. It takes from one to five years for a cancerous tumor the size of a pinpoint and composed of a million cells to form in the body.[2] It's a sure bet that by the time there is a tumor large enough to be felt, cancer has been actively multiplying and spreading in the body for years. Not a comforting thought as you consider how to beat this stuff, but a fact you must be aware of as you consider your treatment options.

Cancer is not just one disease, but many. From the cancer family tree hang the names of as many as 250 related diseases that can originate in any cell of the body. Different types show somewhat different characteristics, but all forms of cancer have two things in common: (1) They consist of abnormal cells that reproduce in an uncontrolled manner after their kind, and (2) they spread, invading healthy tissue in the body.

Our bodies begin as a single cell at conception. From there, through a process of cell division, they take shape. Preexistent cells divide into two new ones, resulting in "daughter cells" that are (or should be) exact duplicates of the original cell. Each comes fully equipped with a genetic code that tells it exactly what to do and exactly how to do it, in order to play its part in bringing about and maintaining the "you" that you're designed to be.

The adult human body is a wondrous collection of trillions of cells, functioning in finely tuned harmony to maintain life. In his book *The Body Is the Hero*, Ronald Glasser, M.D., described the synergism of our bodies as "a great movable city, made up of a trillion individuals all with different skills, yet working together. It has its own ventilation and sewage systems, its own telephone and communications network, a billion miles of interconnecting highways and side streets, a system of alleys, its own super-markets and factories, disposal plants and heating units. All it needs is a few basic raw materials to be brought in."[3]

Somewhere along the line, something happens to alter chemically the genetic programming of a normal cell, disrupting its harmony with the rest of the body. According to the observations of Dr. Otto Warburg—two time Nobel Prize winner for his work with cells—cancerous cells have lost all of their genetically programmed instructions. They no longer know how to contribute properly to the body of which they're part. They retain only the useless property of growth.[4]

If left unchecked by the body's immune system, which is designed to protect it from foreign invaders and mutant cells, a single cancerous cell will multiply independently and out of control. Some of the resulting cells will gather to form localized tumors. Others will be carried by the bloodstream or lymphatic system to different parts of the body. Those that survive begin to form outpost colonies or secondary tumors, referred to in medical terminology as *metastasis.*

Dr. Warburg discovered that cancerous cells are not only damaged in their chemical makeup, but in their means of utilizing energy. They no longer metabolize oxygen as normal cells do to provide energy for their vital processes, but feed on the fermentation of glucose. As cancerous tumors attach themselves to organs, the tissues involved become oxygen starved—essentially fermented. The tumor grows, the vital functions of the organ shut down, and death follows.

WHAT CAUSES CANCER?

As I sit at my computer working on this chapter, thirty books written by various doctors and researchers lie strewn across the top of my desk. Beneath it, stuffed into file folders that fill a large cardboard box, are the articles and clippings of another host of experts. If you were to ask these folks to compile a list of things that have been linked to the cause of cancer, you'd get something that looked like this:

Exposure to . . .
- toxic chemicals in automobile exhaust
- toxic chemicals in secondhand cigarette smoke
- toxic chemicals in industrial air pollution
- toxic chemicals transferred to embryo from parental exposures/diet
- radiation from X-rays
- radiation from excessive exposure to the sun
- radiation leaking from nuclear power plants
- radon gas emitted naturally from our soil
- electromagnetic radiation from high-voltage power lines
- virus-like, parasitic bacteria known as Progenitor Cryptocides

Consumption of . . .
- high amounts of fat and protein from meat and dairy products
- pesticides that have saturated our food chain
- preservatives used in food to extend shelf life
- drugs
- excessive amounts of caffeine

♦ toxic chemicals in drinking water
♦ tobacco products
♦ excessive amounts of alcohol
♦ estrogen hormone
♦ large amounts of cooked or over-processed foods

Lifestyles high in . . .
♦ chronic stress
♦ unresolved conflict

Although not exhaustive, this list nonetheless presents a clear message we must not miss. Truth be known, most cancer is the byproduct of our modern-day lifestyle; the result of choices we've made, individually and corporately, that have had significant repercussions on our health. Dr. Ernest H. Rosenbaum, M.D., among other things the chief of oncology (the study and treatment of tumors) at French Hospital and Medical Center in San Francisco, wrote, "It appears that our affluence—our 'good' life—is the major contributor to the high death rates we have from cancer, as well as heart disease, stroke, emphysema, and obesity."[5]

Open any book or read any text that deals with cancer, and you can arrive at no other conclusion. The great mystery disease of modern humans, the number-two killer moving quickly toward number one, is in large part a nightmare that we've brought on ourselves. We are, in effect, poisoning ourselves to death.

True, for some of us who now have the disease, there were cancer risks in our lives over which we had little or no control. Perhaps, like me, you come from a family history that includes a genetic predisposition toward developing the disease. Even so, your fate was not set in cement. Avoidance of the other risk factors would have been prudent. As the scientists and researchers behind Prevention Magazine Health Books observe, *"80-90% of all cancers are the result of things we do to ourselves.*"[6]

Patrick Quillin, Ph.D., concurs, pointing toward diet as the chief culprit:

> New estimates say that 90 percent of all cancer is environmentally caused and hence preventable. Environmental factors include foods, pollutants, sunlight, tobacco, etc. Of these environmental factors, nutrition (diet) is probably the most important. A conservative estimate states that 30-60 percent of all cancer is nutrition-related. The U.S. has 500 percent more breast and colon cancer than other areas of the world, and much of this dubious distinction is caused by poor nutrition.[7]

Cancer is not, as some people think, "a thunderbolt of fate, striking at random with no cure or cause."[8] There is a cause-and-effect relationship between the environment we've created—the lifestyles and diets we've chosen—and the health problems we're experiencing as a country. When it comes to identifying the chief cause of cancer, we have met the enemy and he is us!

Now I'm not saying all this in an attempt to make you feel guilty or depressed, as if you're somehow a failure in life. You must remember that I am in the same boat as you, a "cancer cousin" dealing with the health consequences of my own choices. Coming from a family history of breast cancer, I was aware of my increased risk. In light of that, I breast-fed my babies, stayed away from coffee and alcohol, and did all that I knew to do at the time. What I didn't know, however, was the link between cancer and the typical American diet. Unfortunately, cancer does not wait for its potential victims to become educated. In my ignorance I gave it an open door to develop in my body.

Wallowing in guilt does none of us any good, but neither does maintaining a naive ignorance that we've played no part in bringing it on ourselves. I remember being assured by my doctors that my cancer was in no way a reflection of something I'd done. According to them, the degeneration of my body into disease was nothing more than a chance occurrence without rhyme or reason—"fate," they called it. But in their attempts to make me feel better by seeking to remove me from responsibility, they did me a great disservice. For when I believed that the onset of my cancer was something over which I had no control or responsibility, I also believed that there was nothing I could do to help my body reverse it. Nothing, that is, other than to subject myself to surgery, radiation, and chemotherapy—"the big three" of modern medicine's therapies against the disease. Had I ultimately bought into the philosophy of "no-fault" cancer, I would have crawled back into my bed and waited for death to arrive, after eventually being told that "the big three" could no longer help me.

❖   ❖   ❖

POINTS TO PONDER

Cancer is a disease of civilization.
It is the end result of health-destroying living
and eating habits, which result in biochemical
imbalance, and physical and chemical
irritation of the tissues.[9]
—Paavo Airola, Ph.D., *How to Get Well*

God has made a universe of moral and material law;
when we break the laws,
we break ourselves upon the laws.
We will reap the consequences in ourselves.[10]
—Richard O. Brennan, M.D.,
Coronary? Cancer? God's Answer: Prevent It!

❖   ❖   ❖

A SYSTEMS FAILURE

Would it surprise you to know that every person has some amount of cancerous cells in his or her body? It only makes sense, for people are regularly being exposed to negative assaults from physical surroundings, aside from the stress of modern-day life and the degenerative processes introduced by the typical American diet. Fortunately, our Creator has given us a built-in, fully integrated defense system, designed to protect and keep us in peak performance. However, if this God-given system becomes weak or dysfunctional, our bodies become vulnerable to takeover by mutant cells—otherwise known as cancer.

Your Immune System

Each of us plays host to an army of white blood cells, known as the immune system—one part of our overall defense system. When cells go bad or foreign agents enter our bodies and threaten to kill us, this army springs to action in a search-and-destroy mission. However, if the body's immune system is weak, cancer is able to gain a foothold.

Virginia Livingston-Wheeler, M.D., author of *The Conquest of Cancer,* wrote,

> Cancer is a disease of the immune system. Or more accurately, it is a disease of a weak immune system. Your immunity must drop to a very low level before cancer can grow, and when it drops to an extremely low and weak level the cancer cells start to spread. Your body has no defense against them, or what small defense it has is not enough.[11]

Dr. Wheeler goes on to observe that "the ability of your immune system to successfully prevent [or in our case, reverse] cancer is directly dependent on your state of nutrition." In other words, diet has a great deal to do with the strength and well-being of our immune system, which in turn has a great deal to do with how well our bodies are able to fight off the occurrence and spread of cancer cells.

Your Liver

Along with the immune system, we come equipped with a mechanism known as a liver. And what a mechanism it is! Besides some 260 other jobs it performs, the liver pulls extra duty as part of the integrated defense system. Not only does it help to keep the immune system strong through its essential role in digestion and assimilation of nutrients from food, but it also serves as a filtering system that removes harmful substances from the blood system that might otherwise do great damage.

Max Gerson, M.D., pioneer in the field of metabolic (nutritional) therapy against cancer, points out the liver's vital importance to the war effort: "To remove the underlying cause and accomplish the cure of cancer means the re-establishment of the whole metabolism, especially of the liver . . . it is the filter for the entire digestive apparatus . . . the liver is the most important organ for our detoxification."[12]

Harold Manner, Ph.D., professor of biology at Loyola University in Chicago, adds these thoughts about the importance of the liver in the battle with cancer:

> There is absolutely no doubt that liver dysfunction is a concomitant phenomenon of cancer. (In other words, where there's cancer, it's a sure bet it was preceded by a poorly functioning liver.) As one of the body's chief organs for the elimination and conversion of toxic substances, the livers of cancer patients have become clogged with many

of the poisons they were meant to eliminate. . . . Cancer can be reversed and controlled only if we regenerate the liver. Fortunately for us, the liver is the one organ in the body capable of regenerating itself. We must immediately institute a program of purification.[13]

Our livers deserve special care and attention. Unfortunately, the typical American diet is counterproductive to liver health. "The foods of the modern diet, especially meats, fried foods, refined oils, and foods with chemical additives weaken the liver," writes nutritionist Ann Wigmore.[14]

Your Colon
One main reason for a dysfunctional liver is a colon that does not allow the waste products from the body to be eliminated effectively. Have you ever had your sewer back up into your house because the system was clogged? In effect, that's what happens when the colon—the body's built-in sewer system—is not functioning as well as it should. Poisonous materials are trapped in the large intestine and reabsorbed back into the bloodstream, only to arrive once again back at the already overloaded liver. As it becomes less and less able to keep up the work of cleaning the blood, the whole body becomes more toxic.

Of the colon, Norman Walker, Ph.D., has written, "Few of us realize that failure to effectively eliminate waste products from the body causes so much fermentation and putrefaction in the large intestine, or colon, that the neglected accumulation of such waste can, and frequently does, result in a lingering demise."[15]

Walker continues, "The fact of the matter is that constipation is the number one affliction underlying nearly every ailment; it can be imputed to be the initial, primary cause of nearly every disturbance of the human system." Perhaps you're thinking just now, "Constipation? I haven't been constipated in years." Research done by Dr. Walker has revealed that constipation of the colon may exist even when movements of the bowel appear to be normal. "If we are eating foods that are cooked or processed, several bowel movements a day are not a sufficient indication that all is well."[16] The colon is notorious for the accumulation of waste materials that, over time, form a rubbery coating on the walls of the colon, keeping it from performing the full spectrum of digestive and waste removal functions it was designed to do. One autopsy done revealed fifty pounds of buildup in a man's colon. Yuck! Most of us probably won't have it that bad, but any buildup is harmful. As a result, the body begins to degenerate.

WHAT TREATMENT STRATEGY MAKES THE MOST SENSE?

By now you're seeing that there is a domino effect in the body—one thing leading to another—allowing for the growth and spread of cancerous cells. The typical American diet of cooked or processed foods, low in fiber and high in fat, can lead to a congested colon and/or dysfunctional liver, which can lead to a weakened immune system, which can lead to cancer. It's obvious that cancer is a "systemic" problem, the result of malfunctions in several individual systems within the integrated body system that are designed to work together to protect us and keep us healthy.

Considering this, the sort of treatment strategy that makes the most sense (at least to this layperson's mind) must ultimately work to restore and rebuild the malfunctioning systems in the body that allowed cancer to grow and spread in the first place. I'm not alone in that opinion.

Earlier I quoted Dr. Max Gerson, pioneer in the field of metabolic (nutritional) therapy against cancer. The

Dr. max Gerson - nutrition in treatment of cancer

world-famous Dr. Albert Schweitzer once said, "I see in Gerson one of the most eminent geniuses in the history of medicine."[17] Concerning the treatment of cancer, Dr. Gerson wrote in *A Cancer Therapy*, "There should be a treatment applied which will fulfill the task of totality in every respect, taking care of the functions of the whole body in all its different parts, thus restoring the harmony of all biological systems."[18]

In other words, treatments aimed only at killing cancer cells or removing existing tumors treat the symptoms of a malfunctioning body, not the body itself. They leave the body system to continue in disrepair (worse for the treatment), allowing for the potential of more cancer to appear at some point in the future. Dr. Patrick Quillin observed, "Many people who do have their cancer medically arrested often experience a new onset of cancer later."[19] A report in *Cancer and Diet* published by the East West Foundation pointed out that in a "British study of women under the age of 30 who had microscopic foci of breast cancer removed, it was found that 25 years later 80% had died of their original disease, despite the fact that their original tumors had been tiny and had been completely removed!"[20]

It's a fact that 75 percent of the people who have been calling me since we've launched our HealthQuarters organization are ones for whom cancer has recurred. Thinking they'd conquered their disease through surgery, radiation, and/or chemotherapy, they're stunned and upset by the fact that not only has it returned, but it's spread to new areas of their bodies.

Surgery, radiation, and chemotherapy—although considered standard procedures for modern-day cancer treatment—do nothing to restore the body's own protective organs and functions in order to keep cancer from returning. They may work to retard the original growth of cancer, or even send it into remission, but they do nothing to remedy its systemic causes. Of these three, none works to cleanse the colon and detoxify the liver. Radiation and chemotherapy actually add to the problem of toxic overload. None works to strengthen the body's immune system. Radiation and surgery are well known to weaken it; chemotherapy is notorious for devastating it.

As the author of *The Conquest of Cancer* stated, "The drugs and chemicals introduced into your system are so toxic, so deadly to cells and tissues, that while they may be doing some good against the cells of a tumor, they are most assuredly weakening your immune system simultaneously."[21] Harold Harper, M.D., observed that "the use of radiation or poison (chemotherapy) in the effort to get at the actual malignant cells is the equivalent of turning a blow torch on a wart."[22]

Used in combination, these therapies can lead to serious immune system collapse. It happened to me. Shortly after my mastectomy and being put on chemotherapy, I was given a two-week course of radiation aimed at destroying three of the tumors that had developed near my backbone. As a result, I wound up flat on my back in the local hospital with a severe case of pneumonia that brought me within a whisper of heaven.

Mine was not an isolated incident. As Dr. Livingston Wheeler wrote, "Irradiation (radiation therapy) and chemotherapy patients often have their immune systems so disrupted that they contract infectious diseases, such as pneumonia, from which they die before the cancer has a chance to kill them."[23]

In defense of "the big three," however, there do seem to be important roles for them to play in the total picture of cancer therapy. In the case of surgery, there are circumstances where the tumor is huge and/or rapidly growing. Cutting it out of the body may be the best "first move" in an overall strategy to get an advantage against the disease. Dr. Wheeler observed that "when you have a tumor of billions of cancerous cells multiplying frightfully fast, you are asking a lot of the immune system to 'catch up' after the cancer has been decimating your own cells for months or even years." In other words, surgery can give your body's own defense system a leg up, a fighting chance. Surgery can help "reduce the number of men in black hats."[24]

It is also acknowledged that there may be instances when a limited course of radiation or chemotherapy could serve as the best "first move" in an overall cancer battle plan. Dr. Kurt W. Donsbach wrote, "There is a place, of course, for surgery or careful and selective radiation, and at times and in certain forms of extremely malignant and fulminating (explosively growing) cancers, the extremely careful use of chemotherapy."[25]

"Nowadays, that's about all we see around here," my oncologist's nurse was heard to say. "By the time most people realize they have cancer, it's already growing pretty rapidly."

Having experienced the world of cancer therapies from the receiver's side, it is this layperson's opinion that "the big three" are radical procedures to be used in crisis situations—not unlike an animal chewing off its leg in order to free itself from a trap. They are invasive, destructive, and potentially life threatening—yet there are times when such drastic tactics are necessary in order to get the advantage on an aggressive enemy. In my own situation, I have no doubt that I would not be around today except by the early and aggressive application of surgery, radiation, and chemotherapy.

At the same time, I also believe that had I not eventually turned to the process of detoxification and rebuilding—otherwise known as nutritional therapy—I would be dead. As Dr. Donsbach pointed out, "None of these modalities [surgery, radiation, chemotherapy] are effective in restoring health, they are merely suppressive and at times help to take a load off of the natural immune system of the body."[26]

It seems clear that if a cancer warrior is going to have any hope of ultimately conquering cancer and winning back health, a very aggressive process needs to be undertaken to reverse the chronic degeneration of the body of which cancer is but a symptom. It all comes down to changing the body's toxic chemistry through the metabolic processes of detoxification and diet—and the sooner the better.

"I am more than ever convinced," wrote Dr. Gerson before his death, "that bio-chemistry and metabolic science will be victorious in healing degenerative diseases, including cancer, if the *whole* body or the *whole metabolism* will be attacked and not the symptoms."[27]

The next three chapters present the details of the metabolic nutritional approach I took to regenerate my own failing system. This process is referred to in various writings and contexts as nutritional therapy, diet therapy, metabolic therapy, natural hygiene, or ortho-molecular medicine. No matter what you call it, the underlying emphasis is the same—restoring the body's own God-given ability to ward off degenerative disease and heal itself.

Take a look at what worked for me. Perhaps you will discover methods that will work for you. Although no one can offer a guarantee, there are *always* possibilities.

❖   ❖   ❖

POINTS TO PONDER

*What if cancer is a systemic, chronic, metabolic
disease of which lumps and bumps
constitute only symptoms?
Will this not mean that billions of dollars*

*have been misspent and that the basic premises
on which cancer treatment and research
are grounded are wrong? Of course it will,
and in decades to come a perplexed future generation
will look back in amazement on how current medicine
approached cancer with the cobalt machine,
the surgical knife, and the introduction
of poisons into the system and wonder
if such brutality really occurred.*
—Harold W. Harper, M.D., and Michael L. Culbert,
How You Can Beat the Killer Diseases

*One can only hope and pray that more and more doctors
will come to see the wisdom in looking beyond surgery,
chemotherapy, and radiation to the wisdom of the ages
and nutritional approaches to reverse the cellular
disturbance which has invaded the body of the cancer
patient. . . . Cancer arises from the poisoning of the cells.*
—Richard O. Brennan, M.D.,
Coronary? Cancer? God's Answer: Prevent It!

*Of course, food as medicine usually affects
the body much more slowly than modern drugs.
But in the end it can be safer and more thorough;
it works by removing the cause of the illness,
whereas most drugs merely relieve the outer symptoms.*
—Ann Wigmore, *Hippocrates Diet*

III

Principle Two—
Cut Off
Enemy Supply Lines

I arrived at her home and was invited into her office, lined with books and bottles. "I'm not going to lie to you," she said. "I've read the results of your blood test and you're a mess. I want to help you, but you must understand that there are no guarantees. Cancer is a degenerative disease and as such can be reversed, but it's hard to say how your body will respond. It depends mostly on the condition of your liver and how well you can restore its full function. What I'm going to recommend for you will not be easy. It's going to demand that you be ruthless with yourself. You're in bad shape internally, not only from the cancer and the effects of chemotherapy, but from thirty-five years of eating the typical American diet, which has provided conditions in your body for the development of cancer in the first place."

So began my introduction to the world of nutrition and nutritional therapy. The concepts that my nutritionist set before me that day were quite overwhelming. I had always thought I was eating a good, healthy diet. What I thought I knew about eating right was crushed by the weight of my ignorance. Yet in my heart and mind, feelings of hope were being renewed. She made no promises, yet the things she said about fighting cancer nutritionally made sense. And I would be taking personal responsibility for my own therapy. I was being empowered to take charge in my own fight toward health. That felt good.

"So, what do you know about nutrition?" she asked.

Mention the word *nutrition* in a room full of typical Americans and most of us will nod our heads as if we have full knowledge about the subject. Ever since we were old enough to sit behind school desks without spilling our finger paint, we have been taught about the "four basic food groups." There's the milk group, the meat group, the vegetable and fruit group, and the bread and cereal group. We were told that these need to make up each meal of our day (or at least our combined daily intake) for proper balance and nutrition. For years we've accepted this organizing scheme as dietary gospel.

However, in the years since 1956, when the U.S. Department of Agriculture began to promote these basic food groups as dietary guidelines for all Americans, questions have been raised. Nutrition scientists and concerned medical doctors have been documenting a growing body of scientific evidence that we Americans have been eating ourselves into early graves.

For instance, consider an eight-page report on diet and nutrition published in the May 27, 1991 edition of *Newsweek* magazine, thirty-five years after the advent of the four basic food groups. It was noted that "our rates of heart disease and some cancers, particularly of the breast and colon are among the highest in the world."[1] The culprit? Too much fat and not enough fiber in our diets. And where does all this fat come from? Primarily the meat and dairy products that we've come to consider as daily essentials based on the "four basic food groups" philosophy.

"Japan offers the starkest example," continues the

report. "The traditional Japanese diet is the direct opposite of ours: typically they eat rice, vegetables and a little fish, while Americans put a big portion of meat in the center of the plate and add a few french fries. Consuming only about a quarter as much fat as we do, and far more carbohydrates, the Japanese live longer than anybody else in the world. That is, until they move here." Quoting Dr. Peter Greenwald, director of cancer prevention and control at the National Cancer Institute: "The Japanese in Japan have one fifth or one sixth the rate of breast cancer that we do. When they move to Hawaii, the rate goes up."

Dietary fat has been linked to many more forms of cancer than just those of the breast and colon. Based on medical studies, Charles B. Simone, M.D., of the radiation therapy department at the University of Pennsylvania, indicates that the mouth, esophagus, stomach, liver, gall bladder, pancreas, ovaries, prostate, kidney, rectum, pharynx, endometrium, thyroid, bladder, and uterus are just a few of the many body parts prone to cancer arising from diets high in animal fat.[2]

It is a well-documented fact that when other countries begin to adopt the typical American diet, the health of those nations suffers. Professor of nutrition at New York University, Marion Nestle said, "I've been in Mauritius, Cuba and Hungary, three completely different countries, advising their governments on nutrition education. People in all three countries are starting to imitate our diet, they're eating more animal fat and dairy products, and their rates of disease are skyrocketing."[3]

How does eating a diet heavy in meat and dairy products contribute to cancer? One factor concerns the bacteria in the digestive system that help to digest food. Simply put, there are good bacteria and there are bad. In the process of digestion "dietary animal fat substantially increases the number of anaerobic bacteria [the bad kind], which produce carcinogens," wrote Dr. Simone.[4] *Carcinogens* are cancer-causing chemicals. The longer they stay in your system, the greater the cancer-causing impact. The typical meat and dairy diet not only increases cancer-causing agents in the body, but it does little to help speed them through the system because of its low fiber content.

John Robbins, who turned his back on fame and fortune as heir to the Baskin-Robbins ice cream dynasty by becoming a health advocate, wrote,

> Without it [fiber], waste gets blocked up, and the length of time your food takes to pass through your colon is greatly increased. This is particularly true if your diet contains animal fat, because animal fats are solid at body temperature. They clog up your intestines just as grease clogs up drains. . . . The longer transit time produced by low-fiber diets provide more opportunity for the bowel walls to reabsorb the toxins the body is trying to eliminate.[5]

Another thing about fat in meat and dairy products is that it "is the most likely storage facility of pollutants from our environment." Dale and Kathy Martin point out in their book *Living Well*, "As we eat upward on the food chain, from root vegetables to grains, fruits, leafy vegetables, vegetable oils, and fats, the concentration of pesticides and other chemical pollutants gradually increases. Dairy products give us a 250% increase of pollutant concentration over leafy vegetables and a 1,500% increase over eating root vegetables." With the consumption of red meat, fish, and poultry, the percentages already cited double.[6]

Fat is the storage place of all the production chemicals that are being put into animals to make them grow bigger and faster. By eating their meat, you and I ingest concentrated amounts of hormones, antibiotics, and other agents that do harm to our own systems.

Bottom line: *Dietary fat from meat and dairy products is bad news!*

In the same week that the *Newsweek* article appeared across the country, *U.S. News and World Report* published a piece on diet and nutrition. They reported that in addition to the dangers of animal fat in our diets, scientific studies are also showing significant evidence that "animal protein (not just the fat) from any source, even dietary do-gooders like poultry and fish, could increase the risk for heart disease, colon cancer, breast cancer and osteoporosis." Quoting T. Colin Campbell, professor of nutritional biochemistry at Cornell University: "Excessive animal protein is at the core of many chronic diseases."[7]

This, however, was not new news. For years the nutritional science community has been aware of the link between high protein diets and cancer. In 1974 Paavo Airola, Ph.D., observed that "the cancer incidence is in direct proportion to the amount of animal proteins, particularly meat, in the diet. . . . Protein eaten in excess of the actual need cannot be properly digested or utilized and acts in the body as a poison and carcinogen. In addition, overconsumption of protein taxes the pancreas and causes chronic deficiency of pancreatic enzymes, which are required for proper protein metabolism."[8]

With all this negative information about the consumption of animal products, you may be wondering if you ought to become a vegetarian. Let me speak to that in the next chapter. For now it's pretty obvious that for the reasons addressed above (carcinogenic bacteria, low fiber, concentrated pollutants and production chemicals, and high protein) meat and dairy products have a lot of strikes against them.

Even the design of the human anatomy points to this conclusion. The human intestine is long and bumpy, whereas the intestine of carnivores, a tiger for instance, is short and smooth. Ingested animal flesh, which ferments at body temperature, is quickly digested and passes through the intestine of a carnivore, but gets slowed down and tends to rot in the intestine of a human being. This sets the stage for a number of health problems. Our bodies just aren't designed to digest meat effectively.

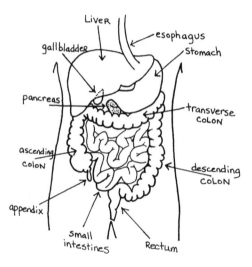

The shelves in my personal library are lined with books and periodicals that decry the evils of the standard American diet (SAD for short), which was based largely on the four basic food groups having equal standing in a "well-balanced" diet. The majority of these works are written by level-headed people—mainly medical doctors and scientists. I could go on and on quoting studies and authorities on the foibles of the typical American diet. If I did you would realize the huge role that politics and money play in compounding our dietary problems. Let me offer just one "for instance" and leave it at that.

Milk is the most political food in the United States.

You and I, whether we like it or not, are in the milk production business. Our taxes go to underwrite the dairy industry "to the tune of almost three billion dollars a year . . . 342,000 dollars every hour to buy hundreds of millions of dairy products that will in all likelihood never be eaten."[9] The government buys dairy surplus to keep production going, letting it rot in storage at a cost of $47 million annually. Millions more are spent by the National Dairy Council every year to get us to drink their product and help reduce their huge surplus. We've all grown up assuming that their commercials were giving us solid facts, that cow's milk makes our bones strong by providing the calcium that our bodies need.

But, in the excellent book entitled *Fit for Life*, Harvey and Marilyn Diamond point out facts that the National Dairy Council would just as soon you not know about their products. "It is important to understand calcium's role in the human body," they write. "One of its main functions is to neutralize acid in the system. . . . All dairy products except butter are extremely acid-forming. . . . The irony is that people are consuming dairy products for calcium, and the existing calcium in their systems is being used to neutralize the effects of the dairy products they are eating."[10] In other words, consuming dairy products for calcium's sake is a "two steps forward, three steps back" proposition. It makes better nutritional sense to get your calcium from raw nuts, seeds, fruits, and vegetables. The very fact that you may find this thought a bit hard to swallow is a tribute to the awesome power of advertising.

The point is this: Most of us don't really know much about the food we put into our bodies. We know mainly what TV commercials and food-industry-related interest groups want us to think. Dale and Kathy Martin observe,

Cancer of the colon looms directly behind lung cancer as the second-ranking, up and coming, cancer in this country. Yet Americans, for the most part, have been unable to recognize the cause and effect relationship between eating the typical American diet and suffering the all-American ailments, many of them terminal. Instead, thanks to heady advertising campaigns from the American Dairy Association, the American Beef Council, and the like, Americans are convinced that dietary choices really are not proven contributors.[11]

We've come to believe that beef really is real food for real people, that chicken and fish are healthy alternatives, and that milk (and associated products) really does do a body good.

But when you're fighting cancer, *it's time to get the facts about what you're putting into your body.* It's time to seek the counsel of a nutritionist or metabolic-nutritional physician who truly specializes in nutrition, or what is sometimes referred to as "third line medicine." (I'll say more about this in chapter 7, "Carefully Select Your Professional Help.") Remember this, *every time you visit the local supermarket your grocery list has the potential to be a great ally in your war on cancer, or an ammo list for your enemy!*

With different words, but along the same lines, my nutritionist introduced me to my need for nutrition education. By now you're asking yourself, as I certainly did, "So what can I eat?" I wondered if I would ever eat again!

In the next chapter I'll outline the dietary guidelines I adopted in order to help rebuild my body's ability to fight cancer for itself. I won't kid you, it was hard. I had to make significant changes in my diet. I was in no position to do less. If the nutritional approach was going to work for me, I had to give it every opportunity. I couldn't fudge (pun fully intended).

Now that I'm cancer free, I've been able to be more

flexible concerning what I eat, while still adhering to certain fundamental principles. Along the way I've learned that tastes are acquired, not inherited. They can and do change. And life is still worth living, even if I can't eat everything I would like to. I don't feel in the least deprived of the foods I *thought* I couldn't live without!

More about all that in the next chapter. For now, let me turn to a discussion of what I learned is the *all-important first step* in any effective program of nutritional therapy against cancer.

INTERNAL CLEANSING AND DETOXIFICATION

My nutritionist said, "First thing you need to do is clean out your body." I was about to embark on the first leg of an "out with the old, in with the new" process.

The ultimate goal of the self-administered cleansing program was to boost my immune system so that it could more effectively go to work against the cancer that had taken over my body. Cancer is, after all, a disease of a weak immune system. But in order to accomplish that goal, at least two things had to happen.

As I mentioned in chapter 2, the liver is a vital ally to the immune system in the war on cancer. Not only does it help protect the body by removing toxic substances from the bloodstream that might otherwise cause cancer, but it also activates the enzymes that metabolize the nutrients from food. These nutrients are in turn delivered to every cell in the body, including the cells that make up the immune system. Are you seeing how important the liver is? Its role in the body's war on cancer is of absolute importance. Dr. Norman Walker wrote, "Be careful of your liver. If it breaks down beyond repair, you will be finished with your body and will have to step out of it forever."[12]

The liver uses a substance it manufactures called bile to flush itself of poisons it has accumulated from the bloodstream. The gall bladder is an attached organ that serves as a storage place for bile. If bile flow through the liver becomes hindered in any way, the waste products and poisons it has removed from the blood build up, and its vital functions slow down. This is referred to as a "sluggish liver." Such a condition "probably reflects minimal impairment of liver function. [But] Because of the liver's important role in numerous metabolic processes, even minor impairment of liver function could have profound effects."[13]

According to the authorities in the field of nutritional therapy, cancer is a likely sign that the liver has been functioning poorly for some time. Not only has it been inadequately flushing poisons from the body, its ability to fulfill its other vital role of helping to keep nutrients flowing to the immune system has also been inhibited.

So what causes bile flow in the liver to be hindered? Simply put, diet! More specifically, the typical American diet. "A fiber-poor, mineral-deficient, and refined diet tends to produce solid particles from bile components (gallstones). . . . But before stones are formed, weakening of the liver due to partially obstructed bile flow may occur."[14] So writes Ann Wigmore, founder of Boston's famed Hippocrates Health Institute and author of *Hippocrates Diet*.

The authors of *An Encyclopedia of Natural Medicine* point out, "It is conservatively estimated that 20 million people in the United States have gallstones—nearly 20% of the female and 8% of the male population over the age of 40 are found to have gallstones on biopsy, and approximately 500,000 gallbladders are removed because of stones each year. The prevalence of gallstones in the US has been related to the high fat/low fiber diet consumed by the majority of Americans."[15]

It became obvious to me that if my immune system was to be strengthened to do effective war on my cancer, I needed first to give immediate attention to cleaning and detoxifying my liver and gall bladder. My hope was that the massive doses of chemotherapy I had undergone had not done irreparable damage to these organs.

The second thing I needed to do was to give attention to my colon, the five feet of intestinal tubing known as the large intestine. I learned that it's not unusual to find in the body of the cancer patient (in fact of many Americans) a buildup of toxic waste substances coating its walls. "Common staples of the American diet, such as white bread, cakes, cookies, meat, milk, doughnuts, spaghetti, and overcooked vegetables, are fiber-poor foods that make it harder for the colon to do its job."[16]

In *Colon Health: The Key to a Vibrant Life*, Dr. Norman Walker referred to fiber as our "intestinal broom." Without its bulk in our diets, the kinds of foods we typically eat "leave a coating of slime on the inner walls of the colon like plaster on a wall. In the course of time this coating may gradually increase its thickness until there is only a small hole through the center."[17] So, even in the presence of regular bowel movements, the colon may be encrusted with a thick rubbery substance that has built up over time.

The longer this toxic waste stays in your colon, the more likely it is that poisons are continually being reabsorbed back into your bloodstream. This can lead to nasty consequences. It's like taking the garbage out to the street, letting it rot awhile, then bringing it back in for dinner. Not only does the liver become overtaxed by all these pollutants reentering the bloodstream, but the blood delivers these toxic materials throughout the whole body where they have opportunity to reap disease-producing havoc on our cells.

"In general, we can say that the blood is only as clean as the bowel," wrote Dr. Bernard Jensen in *Tissue Cleansing Through Bowel Management*, "and since the blood circulates through every organ in the body and reaches every cell in the body, toxins in the blood due to a dirty bowel contaminate the entire body. To properly cleanse the body tissue we must start by a thorough cleansing of the bowel."[18] And so along with my liver and gall bladder, my colon needed deep cleaning attention as well. Check with your own nutritional consultant about all of this.

Enemas

I know, I know. With the mention of the "E" word your mind has begun to rebel. Or perhaps you're unfamiliar with the term. An enema is the gentle flushing of the bowel, accomplished by introducing fluid through a device inserted into the rectum. It's not something that most of us enjoy talking about much. I've noticed that the topic of enemas doesn't seem to come up at dinner parties. Workers don't often linger at the water cooler over the details of someone's latest. I bet you can't even remember the last time you saw a report on television about bowel management. "Good morning, America. I'm Charles Gibson . . . and I'm Joan Lunden. Today we have a colon specialist in the studio, who later in this first half hour will be showing us how we can give ourselves enemas in order to clean out the toxic waste that has built up for years in our colons and livers." That'd be a shocker, wouldn't it?!

Nonetheless, a series of well-administered enemas is an *extremely important* way of helping to cut off enemy supply lines in your battle to regain your health and reverse cancer. The enema is an invaluable asset to the cleansing and detoxification process.

Max Gerson, M.D., mentioned in the previous chapter, wrote this about the importance of enemas for the cancer patient: "Inasmuch as the detoxification of the body is of the greatest importance, especially in the beginning, it is absolutely necessary to administer frequent enemas, day and night."[19] His program calls for an enema every four hours for the first several days of treatment.

Other medical-nutritional authorities who deal specifically with the importance of the enema will bring the details of the procedure together in slightly different ways. For instance, one may suggest that you lie on your left side as fluid is entered, while another may recommend a position on your back or right side. The number of times administered each day is another variable. However, concerning the ultimate goal of the process, the experts are all in agreement: cleanse and detoxify the body's vital organs, particularly the colon and the liver.

My own experience began by administering two eight-cup enemas every day. The first was a water purge enema, used to loosen any deposits of toxic buildup existing on my colon wall. A coffee enema followed immediately. That's right, *coffee!* In her book *Healthy Healing*, Linda Rector-Page, Ph.D., explained, "Coffee enemas have become standard in natural healing when liver and blood related cancers are present. Caffeine used in this way stimulates the liver and gallbladder to remove toxins, open bile ducts, encourage increased peristaltic action, and produce necessary enzyme activity for healthy red blood cell formation and oxygen uptake."[20]

Enemas are easily self-administered. After checking various stores, I found the enema kit I needed at Walgreens. No doubt other drugstores sell them. The one I got came complete with a hot water bottle and hook, a hose that attaches to the bottle with a clamp to adjust flow, and a tip that screws onto the hose and is inserted into the rectum.

Here are the steps I followed in giving myself a set of daily enemas, being sure to be as sanitary as possible.

1. Fluid preparation
   - Warm eight cups of distilled water to body temperature.
   - Brew three cups coffee (don't use instant;

don't use decaf). Add five cups of cool distilled water to bring this down to body temperature.

2. Kit preparation

♦ Find a place where you can lie down and suspend the hot water bottle about twelve inches above you. (Using the hook and a piece of shoestring allowed me to suspend the bottle from the handle in our shower enclosure.) If you're tall you may need to lie on the floor outside the stall or design other arrangements.

♦ Fill the bottle with the water.

♦ Screw hose to bottle and tip to hose (tightly).

♦ Allow a trickle of water to escape before clamping the hose, in order to get rid of air in the line.

♦ Apply lubricant to the tip. Make sure your hands are clean first.

3. Body preparation

♦ Lie down on your left side with your hips elevated. (I used a pillow covered with a plastic bag.)

♦ Insert tip carefully into rectum. (This takes practice. Be gentle, but don't give up.)

4. Flow

♦ Adjust flow to comfort.

♦ Take in as much as comfortable, while massaging your abdomen from left to right to move fluid throughout the colon.

♦ Close clip before removing tip.

♦ Lie on your back, then on your right side for two to three minutes each, continuing to massage your abdomen. (Try to hold in the coffee enema for fifteen to twenty minutes.)

♦ Expel, massaging abdomen from right to left.

5. Clean up

♦ Rinse shower stall, hot water bottle, hose,

tip, and plastic cover on pillow with HOT
water.
♦ Sterilize bathroom surfaces with disinfectant
(toilet, floor, etc.).
♦ Put tip in liquid bleach, washing with HOT
water before using again.

Special note: Because enemas tend to wash out the good bacteria in the colon along with everything else, it is important to consume a daily dose of a live bacteria culture known as "acidophilus" in order to help restore your own natural intestinal flora.

Colonics

My nutritionist highly recommended these, although for reasons of modesty I put off going. After my first one, however, I regretted that I had not made them an integral part of my battle plan.

Colonics, or colon irrigations as they are sometimes called, are glorified enemas. They involve several flushings over a specified period of time (typically an hour), administered by a trained technician using a machine that is specially designed for the purpose. The water flow (several gallons administered a pint or two at a time) and expulsion are controlled by the technician and machine. The goal of a colonic is to use repetition to break down and clean out any fecal deposits in the colon that may be encrusted as a rubbery, difficult to remove coating on the colon wall.

In preparation for writing this book, Dave and I both availed ourselves of the colonic procedure just so we could tell you what it's like as you decide whether to incorporate this into your own battle plan. We found ourselves quite refreshed—cleaned out. The machine pumps the water in; your bowel pumps the water and fecal matter back out through a different channel in the same machine.

Through a glass tube in the mechanism, we saw what was being removed from our colons. It's kind of like searching for buried treasure!

Dave plans to go back for a series of colonics just to make sure his colon is completely clean, then have one or two a year for maintenance purposes. That's pretty high praise coming from him. You'll have to decide for yourself whether you'd like to make colonics a part of your own battle plan. It seems to make sense that even if you have colonics, self-administered coffee retention enemas should still be a part of your program. Check with your nutritional consultant about this.

Juice Fasting

In conjunction with the enemas, my nutritionist put me on a fourteen-day juice fast. In case you're wondering, there's nothing magical about fourteen days. It was obvious, however, that my body was in dramatic need of an extended period of detoxification. After the first three days on the fast, my energy grew steadily. I felt great and my hunger had diminished. But I still tried to rest so my body could cleanse itself. The goal of the fast was to work in partnership with the enemas to clean out my liver and intestines, while at the same time providing my cells with a maximum amount of full-potency vitamins, minerals, natural sugars for calories, and amino acids to build protein. Fresh juices are also packed with digestive enzymes. (Stay away from processed juices. Not only are they usually made from moldy fruit and vegetables, but they are also heat processed, killing the enzymes.) Enzymes are important to the process of metabolizing the nutrients from the food we eat. The more enzymes found in the food itself, the less work required by the liver in the digestive process—a very important fact for the cancer patient whose liver is already functioning poorly. (More about enzymes in chapter 4.)

Because freshly made juices may lose as much as 60 percent of their enzymatic power within a half hour's exposure to oxygen, light, and temperature changes, my husband made juice several times each day. For convenience sake, we sometimes put a batch of juice in a vacuum sealed thermos to extend the life of the enzymes. We purchased a Champion juicer, recommended for its excellence in masticating out the nutrients from fruits and vegetables. Most health food stores can order one for you, if they don't already have them in stock.

The two kinds of juices I consumed most often during my juice fast were apple and carrot. Apple juice is "high in malic acid, pectins, and enzymes that act as a bile solvent and liver stimulant."[21] Carrots are high in beta-carotene, a substance that not only has a beneficial effect on the liver and bile flow, but has been shown to have a significant anti-tumor effect. Often I'd blend in a little fresh lemon juice with my apple. Lemon juice is known to have an antiseptic effect on the body.

The local health food store sold us apples and carrots in bulk quantities, which were organically grown so as to avoid as many chemicals as possible. The juice we made was mixed in a fifty-fifty ratio with distilled water, again to avoid all the possible chemicals that cancer patients can't afford to ingest into their already poisoned systems. I stayed away from tap water. In the beginning I bought bottled distilled water. Later, I bought a high-quality water purifier. The best ones have three filters: a pre-filter, a reverse osmosis filter, and a carbon filter.

To this standard program of several glasses of apple and carrot juices throughout the day, several other components were added to complete my juice fasting routine.

First, each day upon waking I would drink a mixture of two tablespoons of olive oil and four ounces of freshly pressed grapefruit juice. Then I would lie on my right side with my right knee to my chest for twenty minutes. This position opened the pathway to my gall bladder, while the olive oil and juice combination helped to dissolve and clean out any stones that might be forming there. My nutritionist warned that nausea could be part of this process. I experienced a bit, but nothing overwhelming. For me it was mild and passed quickly.

This procedure for cleaning the gall bladder is well documented within the field of nutritional therapy. Some experts think it a bit extreme, what with the potential nausea and all. I've heard that some people do get much sicker than I did. I was grateful, though, that my nutritionist was willing to play "hard ball." She pulled no punches. From the beginning I knew that if I was going to beat cancer, I would have to be aggressive. I needed to get my body cleaned out as quickly as possible. No sense in taking it easy while cancer continued to eat away. I didn't have time to spare, and my nutritionist knew it. This was war!

Another thing she had me do was to add one teaspoon of fiber cleanse to my glass of juice, four times a day. This was done to ensure that my small intestine was being cleaned out, along with my colon. I used generic psyllium husk powder.

Third, five times a day I drank half a glass of distilled water mixed with a teaspoon of "green-drink powder" made from a blend of young barley and wheat grasses, chlorella, brown rice, and kelp. The brand I found most palatable was called Kyo-Green. (See chapter 5 for further explanation.) The nutrients and chlorophyll in this powder build blood, oxygenate cells (cancer can't survive in an oxygenated environment), and act as scavengers of free radicals.

You're probably searching your brain bank for what a "free radical" is. I had never heard the term before. Here's the best way to describe a "free radical": They are highly charged chemical substances made in our bodies as the result of normally occurring chemical reactions. They are molecules with only one electron (stable ones have two) that are on the hunt to swipe a balancing electron from another molecule. "Dr. Roy Walford of UCLA has dubbed them 'the great white sharks in the chemical sea of life.' "[22] Dr. Richard O. Brennan likens a free radical to "a convention delegate away from his wife . . . a highly reactive chemical agent that will combine with anything that is around."[23] This thievery is called oxidation (that's right, rusting) and often sets off a chain reaction that can lead to very negative results. "When radicals are made in the body, the high energy is transferred to body tissues and causes extreme damage to them. If not counteracted, this process can lead to the development of cancer of the tissue affected by the radical."[24]

Normally, the body has built-in defense mechanisms against these free radicals to keep them in check. However, cancer is a sign that the scales have been tipped in favor of a radical takeover. Antioxidants (another name for scavengers of free radicals) play the role of mercenaries sent in to kill and destroy. (In chapter 5, "Bring in Reinforcements," you'll find information about additional antioxidants.)

The fourth element of my routine was to add one teaspoon (4,000 milligrams) of vitamin C powder to four out of five of the green-drinks I consumed each day. In other words, I consumed 16,000 milligrams of vitamin C in each twenty-four-hour period. Vitamin C is another excellent antioxidant, besides inhibiting the spread of cancer and facilitating the proper functioning of the body's immune system.

The final aspect of my cleansing and detoxifying process found me brewing and consuming one quart daily of a specific blend of herbal tea known as Jason Winters' Tea. Made up of chaparral, red clover, and an

Oriental spice called "herbaline," it is well known as a blood cleanser. Among other things, it reduced the nausea I experienced as my body began to clean house, dumping stored up toxins into my bloodstream.

WON'T THE JUICE FAST DO THE JOB WITHOUT ENEMAS?

Not unless you want to wind up poisoning your whole body. Dr. Paavo Airola wrote in *How to Get Well,*

> During fasting a huge amount of morbid matter, dead cells and diseased tissues are burned; and the toxic wastes which have been accumulated in the tissues for years, causing disease and premature aging, are loosed and expelled from the system. These wastes are eliminated from the system by way of kidneys, bowels, skin and lungs. But the alimentary canal, the bowel, is the main road by which these toxins are thrown out of the body. Since, during fasting, the natural bowel movements cease to take place, the toxic wastes would have no way of leaving the system, except with the help of enemas. If you fast without enemas, these toxins remain in your colon and are re-absorbed into the system, poisoning your whole body. Your body will try to get them out through other eliminative organs, particularly through the kidneys, which, as a result, will often be overloaded and even damaged.[25]

The type of fasting my nutritionist was assigning me, intending to aggressively clean out years of toxic buildup, cannot be done without also administering enemas. Without them it would have been like taking poison out of one pocket and putting it back in another. The point was to get rid of it altogether.

SUMMARY

So, there you have it, the details of a detoxification process that helped me clean out my body. My nutritionist referred to it as "giving your inner body a bath." Consult with your own nutritionist as to how long you ought to extend your own juice fast and the other details of your program. To help me keep track of all that I needed to accomplish each day, I set up the following schedule:

8:30 a.m.	grapefruit juice with olive oil (brew Jason Winters' Tea . . . sip throughout day)
9:00 a.m.	apple juice with fiber cleanse, plus enemas
10:00 a.m.	green-drink with C powder
11:00 a.m.	apple juice with fiber cleanse
Noon	carrot juice, acidophilus
1:00 p.m.	green-drink with C powder
2:00 p.m.	apple juice with fiber cleanse
3:00 p.m.	carrot juice
4:00 p.m.	green-drink
5:00 p.m.	apple juice with fiber cleanse
6:00 p.m.	carrot juice
7:00 p.m.	green-drink with C powder
8:00 p.m.	carrot juice
9:00 p.m.	green-drink with C powder
10:00 p.m.	apple juice with fiber cleanse

As you can see, this was serious business. It was important that I become educated about the role of nutrition in disease, then work hard to clean out and detoxify my body of the buildup of years of wrong eating. This was something that required discipline and sustained effort. It wasn't something I could approach as an "add on" to an already busy day. Although I've never been one to enjoy living life by a schedule, nor have I ever considered myself particularly disciplined, this process needed to happen.

❖   ❖   ❖

POINTS TO PONDER

Health is a matter of choice, not a mystery of chance.
—Robert A. Mendelssohn, M.D.

Most health problems begin in the kitchen.
—Paul White, M.D.

Very few people know what real health is because most are occupied with killing themselves slowly.
—Albert V. Szent-Gyorgyi,
Hungarian biochemist and Nobel Prize Laureate
who identified vitamin C

While millions of dollars continue to be poured into cancer research, there are others of us who believe that the most effective research is that done by the individual as he examines his own eating and living habits.
—Richard O. Brennan, M.D.,
Coronary? Cancer? God's Answer: Prevent It!

*In the hand of the physician,
nutrition can be the highest and best remedy.*
—Paracelsus (1490–1541), physician and alchemist
who established the role of chemistry in medicine

The doctor of the future will give no medicine but will interest his patients in the care of the human frame, in diet, and in the cause and prevention of disease. . . . The physician of tomorrow will be the nutritionist of today.
—Thomas Edison

IV

Principle Three— Rebuild Your Natural Defense System

w/ diet + exercise

General Manuel Antonio Noriega emerged tired and haggard from the Vatican's diplomatic mission in Panama City. The dictator-strongman of Panama was ready to call it quits. It was time to throw in the towel. He'd had enough.

Only days earlier, military troops from the United States had converged on the tiny country of Panama, intent on Noriega's capture. Evidence had fallen into the hands of top-ranking U.S. government officials that the general had been secretly aiding Columbian drug cartels in trafficking illegal products to the U.S. It was determined then and there that he was to be stopped.

After eluding troops for several days, the slippery Noriega made his way to the Vatican's diplomatic compound where he sought political asylum from his would-be captors. Holed up and diplomatically out of reach of the United States, it looked as if a protracted stalemate would ensue. Nine days went by without a move by either side. The world watched as tensions mounted. How would this situation be resolved? Who would blink first?

Finally on day ten, a worn and weary Noriega gave himself up. A truck full of troops whisked him off to a U.S. military base in Panama City. There he was formally arrested by agents of the U.S. Drug Enforcement Administration.

At first it was unclear as to what had caused Noriega to give up. For all intents and purposes, it looked as if he could have stayed in the compound for weeks, perhaps months, immune from the long arm of Uncle Sam. There he was sheltered, fed, and protected. He couldn't have asked for a better situation.

So what was it that finally made the general fly the white flag? What drove the strongman of Panama to his proverbial knees? Perhaps the secret lay with Monsignor José Sebastian Laboa, senior ambassador in charge of the mission. "From the very start," admitted the Monsignor when interviewed, "I had a plan to create a psychological environment that would convince Noriega to leave."[1] The details of his plan had involved housing his unwanted guest in a small, un-airconditioned room without access to TV, liquor, or weapons. Cut off from news from the outside, without weapons to mount an offensive, and lacking liquor to fuel his passion, the general didn't last long. The good Monsignor had worked his plan to perfection.

There's an interesting parallel between this scenario of conflict and what it means to battle cancer nutritionally. For just as Monsignor Laboa's strategy was to create an environment in which his unwanted guest felt unwelcome and uncomfortable, the strategy behind nutritional therapy is to create the kind of chemical environment in the body in which cancer finds itself unwelcome and unable to survive.

In the previous chapter I introduced you to the concept of cutting off cancer's supply line by detoxifying your body with juice fasts and enemas—step one toward creating the "cancer hostile" environment. In this chapter and the next I intend to fill you in on step two: *rebuilding and maintaining your body's own natural defense system.* This ongoing process involves three realms: diet, exercise, and supplements. In this chapter I'll cover the first two, and in the next I'll cover supplements.

You've been waiting for my answer to the question, "So what can I eat?" Let's start with that.

A "LIVE FOODS" DIET

Dr. Max Gerson wrote in *A Cancer Therapy,* "Cancer develops in a body which more or less has *lost* the normal functions of the metabolism as a consequence of a chronic daily poisoning accumulated especially in the liver."[2] My blood tests verified my poor liver function. I was about to learn a way of eating that would help my liver rest and my body heal.

"The goal at this stage, now that you've gotten a good start on detoxifying your body," said my nutritionist, "is to begin to rebuild healthy cells. Your immune system, your liver, your colon—every part of your body and its fight against cancer—depend on rebuilding healthy cells. However, the key to healthy cells is the unhindered flow of nutrients from the food we eat. The process of metabolism depends on how well your liver is doing, and right now yours needs a break. It needs time to heal and regenerate, which livers *can* do. You must be eating live foods."

You're no doubt asking the same question that I did: "What are *live foods*?"

"They are foods with live enzymes," she explained.

Suppose that tomorrow morning you were to go out to your car only to find that someone had walked off with your spark plugs. Without them your car is dead, right? Well, enzymes do for your body what spark plugs do for your car. Without them, nothing else can happen. They are *"catalysts,"* wrote nutritionist Maureen Salaman, "proteins, of which there are more than two thousand varieties altogether, that play a vital role in every human physical function."[3] Dr. Mary Swope referred to them as a *"life force* . . . in maintaining health and healing."[4]

Enzymes supply the energy for all the biochemical reactions upon which life is built, including the digestion of food. Our bodies have digestive enzymes, which are reactivated by the liver. The impact of a poorly functioning liver on the well-being of the entire body is obvious: reduced enzymatic activity, which leads to poor digestion, which leads to undernourished cells. In such a state, the body's immune system falters, the organs begin to become dysfunctional, and disease ensues.

Fortunately, there are digestive enzymes in the foods we eat. Nutritionist Ann Wigmore wrote, "Nature's plan calls for food enzymes to help with digestion instead of forcing the body's own digestive enzymes to carry the whole load."[5] So what I needed to do was adopt a diet that would take a load off my liver. I needed to figure out what kinds of foods had a lot of enzymes.

Actually, both plant and animal food products have plenty of enzymes in their natural state. The problem comes when humans get hold of them. Cooking and otherwise processing food kills its enzymes and destroys many of it nutrients. Here are some facts to consider:

◆ Heat destruction of enzymes begins at 107 degrees F and is complete at 122 degrees F.[6]
◆ More than 90 percent of the enzymes in milk are destroyed by modern-day pasteurization methods.[7]
◆ About 65 percent of food in supermarkets has been processed (refined) and, thus, is enzymeless.[8]

The bulk of the typical American diet is dead food. In fact, humans in general are the only creatures on

God's good earth who see fit to alter food before eating it, killing the enzymes and many of the nutrients in the process. If the food we buy at the supermarket has not already had the life processed out of it, we ensure its "deadness" by the way we prepare it for the table. We bake, barbecue, boil, braise, brew, broil, char, fricassee, fry, microwave, sauté, scald, simmer, stew, toast, or otherwise kill the live enzymes in most of our food before we invest it in our bodies. The returns, over an extended period of time, of such investments leave our health accounts bankrupt. To be sure, the body has an amazing ability to sustain life even on the "junkiest" of diets. But simply sustaining life is a far cry from producing vibrant health.

Dr. Norman Walker was a health scientist, author, and practitioner. For eighty years he advocated and modeled a lifestyle built upon the principles of nutrition and healthy living, feeding himself "live foods" from his own garden. In 1985 he died at the age of 109. In one of his many books, he observed that "while such food [dead food] can, and does, sustain life in the human system, it does so at the expense of progressively degenerating health, energy, and vitality."[9]

On the other hand, live foods (foods not already cooked or processed) help keep our bodies strong against disease. Ann Wigmore observed, "If food enzymes do some of the work in the act of predigestion, the metabolic enzyme account (those found in your body) can allot less activity to digestive enzymes, and have much more to give to the hundreds of enzyme systems that run the body."[10] When our body's own metabolic enzymes are "freed up" from having to participate in the process of digesting food, they turn their attention to attacking the protein coating of cancer cells found in our bloodstream. This helps our white blood cells identify and destroy these renegades. "The less demand we make on pancreatic enzymes to digest our food intake, the more enzymes there will be to function as part of our immune defense."[11]

Special note: At times you will be cooking some of your food, even though the bulk of your diet should be raw. Use only stainless steel, glass, or ceramic cookware. Elements like aluminum or teflon that have been popularly used on cookware come off in the food over time and build up in your system.

By now you've been rummaging through the food chain in your mind, listing those things that can be eaten raw. Let's see: raw meat, unpasteurized dairy products, fresh fruit and vegetables, whole grains, raw seeds and nuts—humm. Crossing off raw meat (yuck!) and raw dairy products due to what we've already learned about the health consequences of too much fat and protein in the diet (plus the fact that milk produces mucus that cancer thrives on), you can see which foods make up a "live foods" diet. They are plant products rather than animal products.

Going Vegetarian

I know what you're thinking, and you're right. If you adopt this way of eating you'll become one of "those" kind of people: a vegetarian (*shudder*). It is untrue that vegetarians are always long-haired "weirdos" who smell of incense, look like they've never seen the sun, and spend their free time chanting mantras. It is also untrue that becoming a vegetarian is synonymous with becoming an animal rights activist. I like animals as friends, but I have nothing against eating cows, chickens, pigs, and fish—nothing except the unwanted fat, protein, toxic chemicals, pesticides, and growth hormones in the meat as a result of modern-day production practices.

A vegetarian diet can be very satisfying, even for people like me who grew up keeping McDonald's in business. The trick is to recognize the huge variety of plant foods that God put into our world, then work hard at putting them together creatively into appetizing meals. Besides, once you do this, grocery shopping becomes a snap. Most of your time will be spent in the one aisle where they keep all the live foods. No, not the lobster tank! Wrong kind of live food. I'm talking about the produce aisle.

I must admit that making the switch to a vegetarian diet took some doing. I'd be lying if I said it was easy. Not only did I have to change my tastes, but it took creative thinking to bring variety to my new cuisine. However, some parts of the process require less creativity than others. Breakfast, for instance, on the "live foods" diet is a snap. Either a glass of freshly made apple juice with a bit of lemon or a piece of fresh fruit. I continue to eat fruit during the morning as I get hungry. Lunch, too, is easy. Some blend of raw greens and other vegetables made into a heaping mound of wonderfully colorful salad. My husband and I have become connoisseurs of creative salads. Carrot or other freshly made vegetable juices are great afternoon snacks!

Dinner? That's another issue. For the longest time I struggled with what to prepare for dinner that would qualify as live food. Dinner around our house had traditionally been the big meal, a time when things were most often cooked before hungry mouths devoured. To maintain a habit of live foods for dinner, I began to develop my own set of menus. (You'll find them in appendix A.) Granted, some of the items aren't live—baked potatoes, for instance. But I found that keeping my overall daily intake at about an eighty to twenty ratio—80 percent raw foods, 20 percent cooked (or even better, lightly steamed)—worked well.

What About Protein and Calcium?

As I'm writing this book, I've already been swamped with requests for copies of the partially finished manuscript.

People are hearing about my story and asking for input about what I did nutritionally. As diverse as their backgrounds and health experiences are, their questions are the same when it comes to the "live foods" diet. "If I don't eat meat, how will I get protein?" and "If I don't drink milk, how will I get calcium?"

Like most people, I grew up with the idea that humans need to eat a lot of meat in order to be healthy. Somehow the protein in meat got the reputation of being a "super nutrient," able to help otherwise ordinary people leap tall buildings in a single bound. The more animal protein you ate, the stronger you would become and the healthier you would be. Only as I've gotten involved in nutrition via cancer have I learned how terribly misinformed I was. Here's what I've learned.

First of all, our bodies build their own protein from the foods that we eat. Whether animal products or plant products are consumed, our bodies must first break them down into amino acids, which are then used to produce human protein. In other words, you don't automatically get usable protein by eating it. It all depends on how easily the food product is broken down into its amino acid components.

There are twenty-three kinds of amino acids, fifteen of which can be produced in our systems. The other eight—often referred to as the "essential" amino acids—must come from our diets. "If you eat any fruits, vegetables, nuts, seeds, or sprouts on a regular basis, you are receiving *all* the amino acids necessary for your body to build the protein it needs."[12]

No doubt that's as much news to you as it was to me. I always thought that we needed to eat things with a lot of protein in them to get protein. The real key is the amount of amino acids available in the food. Guess which foods are the easiest for your body to digest and contain the greatest levels of utilizable amino acids—animal or plant products? If by now you see where I'm headed and you guessed plant products, you're right.

The following foods from the plant kingdom contain all eight essential amino acids: bananas, beans, brussels sprouts, cabbage, carrots, cauliflower, corn, cucumbers, eggplant, kale, nuts, okra, peas, potatoes, sesame seeds, summer squash, sunflower seeds, sweet potatoes, and tomatoes. Including these in your vegetarian diet will help ensure that your body is getting the necessary amino acids to produce all the protein you need.

The truth is that it is virtually impossible to get a protein deficiency, even on a strictly vegetarian diet. This, however, flies directly in the face of much, if not all, that you've heard about protein. Like me, you've been sold a bill of goods by the meat and dairy associations and those people they've influenced. "You'd better drink your milk and eat your beef," they imply, "or you'll wind up a ninety-seven-pound weakling."

Edwin Moses would argue with that. An Olympic gold medalist who competed in the 400-meter hurdles for eight years without losing a single race, he's a vegetarian. Dave Scott, also a vegetarian, won the Hawaii Ironman Triathlon a record four times. He's recognized as the greatest triathlete in the world. In *Diet for a New America*, author John Robbins described several laboratory studies comparing meat eaters with vegetarians in strength and endurance. The results showed that vegetarians were two to three times stronger. *Stronger!* Imagine that!

On a vegetarian diet your body is able to produce all the protein you need. At the same time you're avoiding all the fat and excessive protein found in animal products, you're adding fiber to your diet, you're likely cutting down on salt intake, and most of what you're eating will help to keep your system alkaline (a subject dealt with later in this chapter). Let me recommend as required reading *Fit for Life* by Harvey and Marilyn Diamond. They have the absolute best chapter I've ever read on protein! It'll really open your eyes.

Okay, okay, you're saying, so I *can* get all the protein I need from a vegetarian diet. But what about calcium? Don't I need "moo juice" to keep my bones strong? Isn't milk the perfect food?

Well, when it comes from mom it is. But what comes from old Elsie the cow, that's another thing. "The human body is remarkably adaptable, but cow's milk simply isn't designed for humans," the Diamonds point out.[13] In fact, "over 98% of the population is lactose intolerant."[14] By the age of three or four most of us have lost the enzyme called lactase that our body uses to break down lactose in milk.

You will recall what was said in the last chapter about what happens in our bodies when we consume dairy products: We are draining our bodies of their calcium stores. Milk and cheese are extremely acidifying in our systems. In order to counterbalance this effect, our bodies compensate by alkalinizing it with calcium from our own bones. A much better source of calcium would be raw sesame seeds sprinkled on our salads. Other great sources of calcium are kelp, dulse, all leafy greens, figs, dates, and prunes.

Note about nuts: Raw nuts, an excellent source not only of calcium but protein as well, are such a concentrated form of these nutrients that they demand a great deal of metabolic energy to digest. In the rebuilding stage, my digestive system needed a break. Therefore, my nutritionist outlawed them from my rebuilding diet. When I finally reached a point where my cancer was gone, they were allowed.

Discovering Food Allergies

In the process of switching to a "live foods" diet, my nutritionist taught me three important rules. The first rule was this: Avoid foods to which you are allergic. Allergic reactions to food will cause the body to produce mucus in the intestines to protect itself. Cancer feeds on this mucus.

What I'm going to say about discovering what you are allergic to may at first sound like voodoo. Both my husband and I were extremely skeptical—and I do mean *extremely!* But after a double blind study we performed for ourselves, and after countless applications of this method with our family, we've become believers.

I'm talking about a self-administered technique for determining food allergies. Actually, it takes more than just you. You'll need a friend to assist you if you decide to incorporate this into your battle plan. The name of this technique is Muscle Response Testing (MRT), also known in some circles as Applied Kinesiology. The concept behind MRT is that our bodies generate a certain type of electrical current. Scientists and doctors have known this for years. A book entitled *Muscles, Testing, and Functioning* by Kendal and Kendall is said to be the standard on this science and can be found in most medical schools.

My nutritionist had me stand with my strongest arm outstretched from my body in a 90 degree angle, palm down. In the other hand I held against my stomach a food item for which I was being tested. She would stand in front of me as I looked over her shoulder, my mouth closed and feet flat on the floor. Using three fingers, she'd press down on the top of my wrist with firm, steady pressure. A strong muscle feels as though it locks when being tested. An undue amount of force is required to overpower a strong muscle. A strong muscle has a spring-like feeling. If my arm muscle was strong that meant that my body was not allergic to the food item I was holding. The electrical circuit in my body had not been disrupted.

On the other hand, a weak muscle gives way when tested and it does so quite suddenly. It's not a matter of wearing down the person's physical strength. Instead, when you apply force to the arm, the person may resist for an instant, but then his or her strength will be broken. It will feel as though he has surrendered. You can move his arm down quite easily.

A weak muscle, of course, means that the food item you've been holding to your stomach has disrupted the electrical circuit that flows through your body. You've been short-circuited. This is a strong indication that you are allergic to this particular food item.

Okay, you're still skeptical. As I said, we were too at first. I finally satisfied my own mind when I performed a double blind study in my nutritionist's office. The previous week I'd kept the list of everything I'd been tested for. I brought that list back in with me and was retested without her remembering what was put on that list the previous week. I wanted to see if perhaps she was unconsciously influencing the results by the degree of pressure being used with differing items. Each item tested just as it had the week before. Then each item was placed in a separate paper bag by my husband while both of us left the room. Neither she nor I knew the contents of the bags, as one by one I held them to my stomach and was again tested. Again, the results matched those of the previous week.

My family and I have found that MRT is a good way to test for food sensitivities to whole foods. In other words, you wouldn't hold a handful of salad to your stomach. You would want to separate its basic elements—lettuce, carrot, cucumber, black olive, tomato, etc. Speaking of tomatoes, I discovered that my body was sensitive to them. Interestingly enough, after a period of time, as I continued to clean out and build up my body, the allergy disappeared. I am now eating things that I haven't been able to tolerate for years, long before I even knew cancer was growing in my body.

Combining Food Right

The second rule that my nutritionist taught me had to do with the order and combinations in which to eat foods.

I had never known that different kinds of food require different kinds of digestive juices and enzymes. Therefore, eating a variety of foods together during a single meal throws the digestive system into chaos, making proper digestion impossible. We've all felt the effects of Thanksgiving feasts on our systems. What results is a mass of putrefying, fermenting stuff stuck in the stomach that the body is working hard just to get rid of. Extraction and absorption of nutrients in an effort to build and maintain healthy cell life is greatly hindered. In fact, "nutrients affected in this way cannot be incorporated into healthy cell structure."[15] The consistent habit of improperly combining our food—a very common practice in the United States—leads to cellular malnutrition.

The whole point of food combining is to eat foods in the same meal that are digested in the same way so as to reap maximum nutritional benefit. Simple food combining guidelines include:

◆ Eat fruit by itself.
   Fruit is a very important kind of food, but
   must never follow something else in a meal. It
   is predigested food, moving right through the
   stomach into the intestines—"except for bananas,
   dates, and dried fruit, which stay in the stomach
   a bit longer."[16] If fruit is eaten immediately after
   another kind of food, it will ferment itself and
   everything else in the stomach.

◆ Eat vegetables and proteins together.

◆ Eat vegetables and starches together.

For more about food combining, let me recommend *Fit for Life* and *Fit for Life II: Living Health* by Harvey and Marilyn Diamond. Perhaps no others in the field of nutrition know more about this science.

Keeping an Alkaline Balance

When food is digested or "burned" by the body, it leaves what is referred to as "ash." Some foods burn down to an alkaline ash, others an acid ash. In *Health Through Nutrition*, Dr. Joel Robbins expounded on the necessity of eating foods that help keep an alkaline balance in our bodies:

> The cells of the body in health are alkaline. . . . The more acid the cells become, the sicker we feel. . . . Our bodies produce acid as a by-product of normal metabolism. Since our bodies do not manufacture alkaline, we must supply the alkaline from an outside source to keep us from becoming acid and dying. Food is the means of replenishing the alkaline to the body. . . . We can remain in health by consuming a diet that is 80% alkaline and 20% acid.[17]

Dr. Robbins went on to point out that, unfortunately, the typical American diet is just the opposite: 20 percent alkaline and 80 percent acid.

"In the healing of disease," wrote Dr. Airola, "when the patient usually has acidosis (over-acidity), the higher the ratio of alkaline elements in the diet, the faster will be the recovery."[18]

Rule number three was to make sure that my live foods diet was selected primarily from alkaline ash foods. This was actually fairly easy. The family of alkaline foods contains most kinds of fruits and vegetables—whether raw, juiced, dried, frozen, or lightly steamed. Interestingly enough, this includes "even the acid fruits such as oranges, pineapples and grapefruit. These are only classified botanically as acid fruits."[19] Once these hit the stomach they become alkaline, that is if they're eaten by themselves as we've already seen that all fruit should be.

"All vegetable and fruit juices are high alkaline," observes Dr. Airola. "The most alkaline-forming are: fig juice, green juices of all green vegetables and tops, carrot, beet, celery, pineapple and citrus juices."[20]

A list of some of the individual members of the alkaline ash family includes, from most alkaline to least: figs, soybeans, lima beans, apricots, spinach, turnip or beet greens, raisins, almonds, carrots, dates, celery, cucumber, cantaloupe, lettuce, watercress, potatoes, pineapple, cabbage, grapefruit, tomatoes, peaches, apples, grapes, bananas, watermelon, millet, brazil nuts, coconuts, buckwheat. Except for millet and buckwheat, most grains are acid-forming. Sprouted seeds and grains become more alkaline.[21]

Here's a list of some of the individual members of the risky acid ash family, from most acid to least: tobacco, drugs/medications, alcohol, salt, coffee/tea, fried meats, herbs/spices/condiments, red meats, fried pastries, fried fruits/vegetables, white meats, sugar/refined grains, dairy products/eggs, overcooked fruits/vegetables, whole grains, some raw fruits and vegetables (cranberries, blueberries, plums, prunes, squash), raw seeds (sesame, pumpkin, squash, sunflower), raw nuts (except almonds).[22]

FATS

My nutritionist recommended a *low* fat diet. Notice that I didn't say a *no* fat diet. Fat is an essential part of human nutrition. Too much fat is cancer causing. The elimination of animal products helps bring our fat intake down to acceptable levels. I had to learn the difference between good fats and bad (carcinogenic) fats. Fats go rancid (rotten) soon after being separated from their source. Fats that have been heat processed are highly carcinogenic. Fats that have been "hydrogenated" have been heat processed. Oils should be unrefined and cold pressed. Extra virgin olive oil is an example of a good kind of fat. Avocados also contain good fat. We learned to make some stuff called "better butter." One cup of canola oil is mixed in the blender with two sticks of butter, then refrigerated. I was allowed to use it sparingly. I didn't use margarine at all. According to my nutritionist, it's only one ion away from being plastic!

IN PRAISE OF FRUITS, VEGETABLES, AND GRAINS

In recent months the U.S. government has taken to heart the pressure it has received from many advocates of nutrition to do away with the "four basic food groups" as dietary guidelines for healthy eating in the U.S. With scientific evidence mounting that meat and dairy products are far less important for human health than are fruits, vegetables, and grains, the folks who spend our tax dollars have come up with a brilliant idea. Knowing that we Americans are notoriously bad about eating things that are good for us, they've developed a federally funded project called "Designer Foods."

Our local newspaper reported, "With a budget of $20.5 million over the next 5 years, its goal is to create a new processed food product (a nutritional milkshake) containing concentrated amounts of the natural cancer-preventing 'phytochemicals' found in plants."[23]

Hey, I have a better idea. Let's divide that $20.5 million amongst all the households in the country and make everyone plant a garden! It's impossible to improve on nature!

❖ ❖ ❖

POINTS TO PONDER

Let food be your medicine,
and medicine be your food.
—Hippocrates, fifth-century doctor
traditionally regarded as the "father of medicine"

*Truly the vegetable kingdom
contains our best medicines.*
—Henry G. Bieler, M.D.,
Food Is Your Best Medicine

*All the nutritional requirements
that the human body has—all the vitamins,
minerals, proteins, amino acids,
enzymes, carbohydrates, and fatty acids that exist,
that the human body needs to survive—
are to be found
in fruits and vegetables.*
—Harvey and Marilyn Diamond,
Fit for Life

*If someone eats what is useful for his health
and avoids other things that may shorten his life,
then he is a man of wisdom and self control.*
—Paracelsus (1490–1541),
physician and alchemist who established the role
of chemistry in medicine

*I believe that millions of people today
can attest to the effectiveness of eating raw,
natural, unprocessed, organically grown food
in the building, repair and maintenance
of healthy, disease-free cells in our bodies.*
—Mary Ruth Swope, Ph.D.,
Green Leaves of Barley

*The coming years will make it more
and more important that organically grown fruit
and vegetables will be, and must be,
used for protection against degenerative diseases,
the prevention of cancer, and more so
in the treatment of cancer.*
—Max Gerson, M.D.,
A Cancer Therapy

It is my view that the vegetarian manner of living,
by its purely physical effect on the human temperament,
would most beneficially influence
the lot of mankind.

—Albert Einstein

❖   ❖   ❖

EXERCISE

Shortly after I was diagnosed with cancer and began chemotherapy treatments, my oncologist began an exercise program for his patients at a local fitness club. At first I was scared to death to go. I'd just had a mastectomy, I still had a stress fracture in my backbone, and I'd been flat on my back in pain for a couple of months. The thought of exercise struck absolute terror in my heart. I was just sure I would either break in half or simply wilt from the pain of physical exertion. The night before I was to attend my first workout, I cried my eyes out.

I started slowly. Very slowly! My first attempts were nothing more than to raise my arms up to shoulder level. From there I graduated to a loose rubber band positioned under my foot that produced a little tension as I pulled the other end to shoulder height. All along, my progress was being monitored by a physical therapist on my oncologist's team. We faithfully recorded the smallest improvements. It took a long time, but eventually I was pumping iron with the men! I attended regularly, discovering in the process two beneficial effects of exercise in an overall cancer battle plan.

The first was psychological. Just being there with healthy people doing healthy things was emotionally nourishing. "When patients realize they can maintain an active lifestyle they are less fearful," my oncologist said. "They have greater hope and greater enthusiasm."

I started seeing myself as a normal person again. Eventually I was keeping up in aerobics class alongside folks who didn't even have cancer. It felt good, like I was human again. I felt more in control of my body. I was actually doing something to improve my health. Every time I went in for a workout (which became three times a week), I would push myself to do one more minute on the bike or add one more repetition to the number of lifts. I was challenging myself and seeing positive results. It was emotionally encouraging to see improvement. In at least one respect, I could see my body making progress. (In chapter 6, "Maintain Morale," I'll say more about the psychological aspects of fighting cancer.)

"Exercise also tends to alleviate a lot of the family's fears," observed my oncologist. "The immediate response of the families of many cancer patients is to try to take care of them, do things for them. That's hard to do when the person is working out at the gym."

In *Getting Well Again*, Dr. Carl Simonton and his wife, Stephanie, wrote about the role of exercise in their own experiences of helping cancer patients overcome the disease:

> We began paying more attention to exercise when we observed that many of our patients with the most dramatic recoveries from cancer were physically very active. Because physical activity appears to be a way of releasing stress and tension, it is also an effective way of changing one's state of mind. As a result, we have developed a program of physical exercise that we ask all our patients to try. We believe that regular exercise provides a way for patients to participate in getting well. . . . When the quality of life improves, so do people's commitments to living and beliefs that they can recover.[24]

The second benefit I experienced was, of course, physical. I was getting stronger and my body was healing. The weight lifting caused my wounded bones to heal, including the stress fracture in my back. My heart and lungs were also getting stronger. I have no doubt that had they not been as strong as they were, I would not have taken chemotherapy as well as I did. In fact, I might well have died in Omaha during the bone marrow procedure. The massive doses of chemotherapy and ensuing struggles to regenerate white blood cells would probably have done me in. My oncologist concurs that the more physically fit the patient, the better able they are to tolerate the chemotherapy treatment.

Besides getting stronger, I found myself with more energy during the day, sleeping better at night, eliminating waste from my body more regularly, and experiencing better blood circulation. Since cancer cells can't survive in an oxygenated environment and healthy cells thrive on it, the increased level of oxygen being delivered through my bloodstream was doing its part in my overall battle against cancer. Then, too, exercise tends to stimulate the immune system. Not only was my workout program helping to produce a fighting spirit in me and making me physically stronger, it was stimulating my defense system to go to war more actively against my cancer.

Should every cancer patient start some sort of exercise program? Here's what Dr. Simonton said:

> While some specialists might consider it [exercise] inadvisable for patients with cancer that has spread to the bone, for those with low platelet counts [the mechanism that assists in blood clotting], or for those with other limiting conditions, we believe that most patients, even those with these special conditions, can maintain an exercise program. Our

primary caution is that they should proceed at a slower pace, recognizing that it is possible to injure themselves, and carefully observe any warning signals of pain or stiffness.[25]

This would be a great day for a walk, wouldn't it?

SUMMARY

Please remember the major points we have covered in this chapter. A live foods diet is important for rebuilding healthy cell life. A person can get enough protein and calcium on a vegetarian diet. It's important on your live foods diet that you identify and refrain from eating any foods to which you are allergic. Also be careful to combine the foods you eat correctly, eating foods together that require the same digestive fluids. Doing this will ensure that your body gets full use of the nutrients. One advantage of a live foods diet is that it helps to keep your system alkaline.

As for exercise, do it! If you don't already have an exercise program, start one. Start slowly, but do start! Write your ideas in the box below.

---

*This is what I'm planning to do
in order to get going on an exercise program:*

V

Principle Four— Bring in Reinforcements

In 1866, after an illustrious career as a Union officer in the Civil War, George Armstrong Custer was promoted to lieutenant colonel of the seventh U.S. cavalry in the regular army. His orders took him west to Kansas where he was to take part under General W. S. Hancock in a campaign against the Cheyenne Indians. After a convincing battle in which the Indian forces were badly crushed, Custer spent the next several years in relative peace.

But in 1876, Custer and his men were once again ordered into battle against the Indians, this time against the Sioux in Montana and Dakota led by Sitting Bull and Crazy Horse. It was to be a two-pronged attack under the command of General A. H. Terry. Custer was to lead one column while Terry led the other, attacking the Sioux in a combined effort for maximum impact. Custer, however, arrived at the agreed-upon rendezvous near the Indian camp on the Little Bighorn River two days earlier than Terry. For whatever reason—most likely a desire to bolster his own ego—he disobeyed orders and formed his own battle plan. The next morning he divided his men into three units and attacked, before reinforcements could arrive. The central unit, led by Custer himself, rode directly into the heart of the enemy camp. Not a single soldier survived.

What has since come to be known as "Custer's Last Stand" holds a lesson for those of us who are battling cancer. In fighting cancer, as in waging war, it is vitally important to the prospect of victory to be able to call in reinforcements when they're needed.

You've just read a chapter that focuses primarily on a "live foods" diet as key to healthy cell life and beating down cancer. Some in the field of nutrition will say that the average person should be able to get all the needed nutrients from such a diet and will not need supplements. The problem is that people who are fighting cancer begin "in the hole" nutritionally. They are not the "average" person with a fully functional metabolic system. Their bodies are malfunctioning—evidenced by the emergence of cancer—and no doubt have been for quite some time. Quite often their liver-gall bladder combination is not carrying out its metabolic functions properly. Certain kinds of necessary nutrients cannot be properly used by the body unless first broken down by bile acids made by the liver and stored in the gall bladder. "Without these bile acids, all fat-soluble vitamins do not get properly absorbed into the blood, resulting in a vitamin deficiency."[1] Various kinds of dietary supplements need to be added to the battle plan in order to supply the body with the nutrients it desperately needs but hasn't been able to get because of poor metabolism.

The following pages contain a list of the various supplements that I added to my own battle plan. I share it with you to familiarize you with what's helped me. It's possible you may need to start taking a number of these, but *please* don't use this list as a blueprint to reproduce automatically. Ask your own nutritionist what sort of supplements you ought to be taking and how much of each, based on the details and circumstances of your own condition.

The object of vitamin and mineral supplementation in the battle against cancer is to rebuild healthy cells, change body chemistry, and reinforce the body's own protective systems. Vitamins and minerals don't cure cancer; they help restore and reinforce the body's own ability to fight off the disease. This is an important fact to remember. Along these lines, Dr. Joel Robbins has observed that "it's the body's action or utilization of the nutrients for healing, not the nutrient's action on the body," that counts.[2] In other words, if the body is already so far gone in disease that it can't utilize what is being put into it, vitamins and minerals will do little good.

It's just as important to realize that "vitamin/mineral therapy and supplementation do not produce results overnight. Vitamins (and minerals) are at the deepest levels of the body processes, and regenerative changes in body chemistry usually require as much time to rebuild as they did to decline."[3] In our fast-paced culture, people typically look for a "quick fix" to their medical problems, something to take—often drugs—to make everything better soon. Reversing degenerative disease, however, is not a quick-fix proposition. It's a matter of an extended period of time spent working to revitalize the entire metabolism and chemistry of a body system that has been heading downhill for perhaps a very long time.

Dr. Max Gerson wrote,

In general, people go to hospitals for operations or serious illness; the family considers them recovered upon their return. This is different with cancer. Cancer is a degenerative disease, not an acute one, and the treatment can be effective only if carried out strictly in accordance with the rules for one and a half to two years. . . . It is not a symptom that is treated, nor a specific disease, but the reactions and functions of the entire body which have to be transformed and restored.[4]

That said, let me introduce you to the reinforcing troops that have come alongside my "live foods" diet to help me win back and maintain my health. Each of them has many more roles in the body than I've listed. I've intentionally kept their job descriptions to a limited focus.

VITAMINS

Vitamins are organic micro-nutrients that work in the body together with enzymes to regulate metabolic processes and convert proteins and carbohydrates to tissue and energy. They keep the body tuned up and functioning at peak performance. Healthy growth, vitality, and disease-free aging are not possible without them. Even though the body needs them in very small amounts, vitamins must be supplied from food. The majority are not manufactured in the body. While some vitamins are fat soluble and can be stored in the body (A, D, E, K), others are water soluble and must be continually replenished (B-complex, C).

Vitamin deficiencies, even if very small, can have a significant effect on the health and well-being of the entire body. Unfortunately, deficiencies are not easily identifiable. Insufficiently supplied cell life can continue to function for some time—albeit at lower and lower levels of effectiveness—until reinforcing nutrients arrive on the scene or the cell dies.

Vitamin A (Emulsified)

Vitamin A is known as an excellent antioxidant, able to go to bat against free radicals in the body that cause cancer. (Free radicals are defined and explained in chapter 3.) It is a fat-soluble vitamin, meaning that it requires the action of bile acids made in the liver in order to be properly absorbed into the blood. Fat-soluble vitamins are also stored by the body and can therefore reach toxic levels. Vitamin A in emulsified form, however, is water soluble. It doesn't need the liver's action in order to be absorbed into the bloodstream, nor is it stored in the body. This is important for the cancer patient whose liver is not functioning properly. Studies have shown that emulsified A can be safely taken in large doses without toxic overload.

Vitamin A is a prime component of a strong immune system, stimulating in particular the lymphocytes (T cells) to fight cancer. It also works to protect the cells that make up the skin and the linings of the many organs and passageways in the body (respiratory tract, digestive tract, urinary tract, reproductive tract). Statistics show that over half of all human cancers start in these tissues known as "epithelial tissue."

Vitamin A is also a key to cell differentiation. To quote Michael B. Sporn, M.D., "Differentiation is the process that makes the cell what it is, that allows it to carry out the normal functions of a cell. When a cell dedifferentiates, those functions are lost, and the cell enters a primitive state. Its behavior becomes similar to that of a cancer cell."[5] Vitamin A helps to ensure that cells grow up and do what they are supposed to.

Beta-Carotene

I didn't actually take this as a supplement. I got plenty of beta-carotene in the carrot juice I drank each day as part of my live foods diet. But I wanted to mention it because of its tremendous benefit to the cancer warrior. Beta-carotene is a very effective agent at stimulating the immune system to protect the body. It is also a powerful antioxidant and free radical scavenger. In fact, it's the most efficient neutralizer of singlet oxygen, a high-energy, very destructive free radical. Like vitamin A, it too is fat-soluble and stored in the body. Unlike vitamin A, it does not reach toxic levels in the body. The liver converts it into vitamin A only as it is needed.

In *How to Fight Cancer and Win*, William L. Fischer noted the following beneficial characteristics about beta-carotene:

> As both a preventative and an active cancer treatment, beta-carotene has been shown to effectively destroy the cancer cell's protective layer of mucus, opening it to the body's natural defense mechanisms. Proponents of beta-carotene predict reductions in the rate of certain forms of cancer for those who regularly include carrots in their diet (up to 80 percent of cancer in the lungs and bronchia, and up to 55 percent in cancer of the colon).[6]

Three cheers for the lowly carrot! It is the most important source of natural beta-carotene on God's green earth. This "commoner" in the cabbage patch has reached kingly stature in the cancer fighting community.

B-Complex Vitamins

Teamwork is something special. It's a finely tuned basketball team that wins the championship or a music group that tops the charts or a medical unit that successfully performs a heart transplant. It's the process in which each individual part adds its special strengths to the others, multiplying the impact of the whole.

The B-complex water soluble vitamins function as such a team. It includes: thiamine (B_1), riboflavin (B_2), niacin (B_3, or nicotinic acid), pyridoxine (B_6), biotin, inositol, para-aminobenzoic acid (PABA), cyanocobalamine (B_{12}), pantothenic acid, and folic acid.

I added the B-complex vitamin team to my arsenal of reinforcements for three reasons: (1) My heart had been badly abused by all the chemotherapy and the B team helps to heal hearts, (2) various members of B-complex work to enhance and stimulate the immune system, and (3) some B vitamins help *inhibit* the growth of cancerous cells and tumors.

Vitamin C
Ah, the big gun! It is a recognized fact that the presence of vitamin C in the body inhibits cancer, and the absence of vitamin C increases cancer risk. It is also a know fact that vitamin C is one of the most potent antioxidants known to science. Patrick Quillin concluded,

> Vitamin C stimulates the immune system to attack the newly sprouted abnormal cells. It is a free radical scavenger, mopping up free radicals to prevent destruction of the DNA. It stimulates the production of interferon, a potent anticancer agent in the body. It blocks the formation of carcinogenic nitrosamines in the stomach.[7]

Another observed characteristic of vitamin C is its ability to inhibit cancer from spreading in the body by neutralizing a certain enzyme produced by cancer cells that would otherwise help the cancer metastasize.

Linus Pauling, Ph.D., a two-time Nobel laureate who has spent years researching vitamin C's effects, notes that "a high intake of vitamin C is beneficial to all patients with cancer. . . . With the proper use of vitamin C for cancer, we could cut the death rate by 75%. This would be 75% of 650,000 people who die every year of cancer. These are people whose lives could have been extended with the use of vitamin C."[8]

Everyone has heard by now about the extreme value

of vitamin C to the human body. The question is not whether to take it, but how much. Dr. Pauling takes 10,000 milligrams a day (ten grams). How much vitamin C should a person with cancer take? For a time I was taking as much as fifty grams intravenously once a week. That's 50,000 milligrams! Generally, ten to fifteen grams daily of vitamin C is recommended for cancer patients. Check with your nutritionist on what amount would be right for you. It's important to work up gradually to these high levels of vitamin C. Your tolerance will build. I started with one gram four times a day and worked up to fifteen grams daily, in powder form mixed into my juice.

Jonathan V. Wright, a well-known nutrition-minded M.D., wrote, "Considering air, water, and food pollution, which we all are exposed to and which vitamin C will detoxify, not taking extra vitamin C every day is a definite health hazard."[9]

Vitamin E (Emulsified)
Vitamin E, like A, is fat soluble. Therefore, I took it in emulsified form. And like A and C, it is an antioxidant for hunting down free radicals and destroying them. It is also an important immune system stimulant. When vitamin E is teamed with selenium, anticancer properties of both are enhanced. And like vitamin C, E is thought to hinder the production of cancer-causing nitrosamines (powerful compounds) in the stomach and intestines.

MINERALS
Without minerals, vitamins would do us little good. Minerals are the building blocks of life. They are the most basic of nutrients, components of the earth's crust. Minerals allow our bodies to digest food, absorb nutrients, and keep an alkaline pH balance, rather than acid.

My nutritionist had me take a wide spectrum of minerals in liquid suspension form every day to ensure that my body was getting what it needed. Some important minerals also needed to be found in other supplements I was taking.

Copper
The systems of people with cancer have always been found to be deficient in copper. Therefore, I was to make sure that copper was included in other supplements besides the liquid minerals.

Magnesium
Magnesium was another of the minerals I was to pay particular attention to getting in supplements other than the liquid minerals. With all the chemotherapy I'd had, I was at risk of heart failure. Magnesium is known as "one of the heart's best friends," protecting it in many ways and keeping it healthy. It is also a necessary agent in the body for muscle relaxation and the absorption of other minerals.

Zinc
Zinc was one mineral I took in supplement form by itself, along with what I received in the liquid minerals. It is a key component of a vital enzyme in the body known as superoxide dismutase (SOD). Incorporated into this potent antioxidant, zinc becomes a powerful weapon for destroying invasions of free radicals in the body. SOD protects our DNA from free radical damage, which could cause cancerous mutations. It has actually been referred to by some experts as an "anticancer" enzyme.

Selenium
To the list of minerals I was to include in the additional supplements, selenium was added. Much has been written about this trace mineral and its ability to fight cancer. Those who are studying its impact on the human body are saying that it may be one of the most promising weapons in the nutritional battle plan against cancer.

Selenium has shown itself to be one of the more potent anticancer agents available. When teamed with vitamin E, the effectiveness of both against cancer is further amplified. They work together in a potent anticancer, anti-aging system called glutathione peroxidase (GSH). This combination forms a potent antioxidant, and thus, scavengers protect cell membranes from free radical attack. GSH has been likened by some to a miniature police force that seeks out and destroys rebellious cells and free radicals within the body. It is without question an important weapon for the body to ward off cancer. The amounts of vitamin E and selenium in one's diet affect the levels of GSH in the body.

A variety of other properties have been shown to be true of selenium:

◆ It improves the efficiency with which DNA can repair itself.
◆ At high levels it is directly toxic to cancer cells.
◆ It retards the growth of tumors in human breast tissue.
◆ It can deactivate radiation toxicity in the body.
◆ It works to clean the blood from the effects of chemotherapy and liver malfunction.
◆ It is a potent stimulant to the immune system.

So you see how important this trace mineral is to the cancer warrior. Scientists have noticed a direct link between the incidence of cancer and the levels of selenium in the soil in different parts of the country. Where the levels are lower, the population's incidence of cancer is higher.

MISCELLANEOUS TROOPS
EPA-DHA (Fish Oil)
Fat in our bodies tends to encourage the development of

cancer. However, some fats are beneficial. Two of the better known omega-3 fatty acids are active ingredients in fish oil: eicosapentaenoic acid (EPA) and docosahexaenoic acid (DHA). They have been referred to by some biochemists as "wonder" fats in that they actually protect against cancer.

EPA and DHA are known to stimulate the production of prostacyclin, which works toward cleaning up cancerous growth in the body. They also inhibit arachidonic acid byproducts, which can cause cancer. In animal studies, they resulted in significant reduction in the size and weight of breast tumors. In addition to all these things, EPA is known to stimulate the human body's immune system.

Glutathione

I took this amino acid as a supplement. Glutathione functions in the body as an antioxidant, not only going after free radicals but fighting radiation toxicity. It also serves to clean the blood of the effects of chemotherapy and liver malfunction.

Fiber Cleanse

The need for fiber in fighting cancer seems obvious. Fiber helps to establish a clear path for the removal of toxins from the body via the colon. It also has several other properties in the body, including:

- ◆ The absorption and removal of problem-causing substances, including fats, cholesterol, heavy metals, and drug accumulation.
- ◆ Preventing bacteria from degrading cholesterol into deoxycholic acid (a known carcinogen) in the intestine.
- ◆ Increasing the growth of friendly intestinal bacteria.
- ◆ Helping to retain important B-complex vitamins.

Melaleuca Oil

When I returned from Omaha after my bone marrow transplant, a coating of fungus had grown thick on my tongue. Through the cancer fighting grapevine I learned that cancer thrives on fungus in the blood and melaleuca oil is a wonderful antifungal agent. Made from melaleuca trees, it smells and tastes just like turpentine (although I've never really tasted turpentine). I began using a dose of three to five drops three times a day in a swallow of water or juice, sometimes mixing it with green-drink. Holding my nose helped me get it down. I continue to use melaleuca oil once a week to help keep my body free of fungus. My nutritionist was also aware of studies that showed melaleuca oil to be effective against cancer in the bones. It made sense to add this to my battle plan. A common name often used for this substance is Australian tea tree oil.

Green-Drink

In chapter 3, I briefly introduced you to green-drink. There are a number of different brands in powder form on the market. They contain a variety of ingredients, including wheat grass, young barley leaves, kelp, blue-green algae, brown rice, and chlorella. The package of nutrients this kind of concoction delivers to the body is amazing: amino acids, nucleic acids, chlorophyll, minerals, enzymes, vitamin A, beta-carotene, calcium, iron, and potassium. It all works together as a potent blood builder, oxygenator, free radical scavenger, cell builder against disease, and foundation for building protein.

In her book *How I Conquered Cancer Naturally*, Eydie Mae Hunsberger told how she made green-drink from wheat grass she grew in her own greenhouse. Making it yourself out of freshly harvested ingredients definitely ensures getting the greatest benefits. If you'd like to give it a shot, read her book or others written by her mentor Ann Wigmore, founder of the Hippocrates Health Institute of Boston, Massachusetts. As for me, I preferred a powdered form called Kyo-Green mixed with distilled water. Although I tried several of the other brands on the market, Kyo-Green was the one I found most palatable. It was also the one my nutritionist recommended above all the others. One teaspoon taken in a glass of cold water or juice four or five times a day helped to give my body the sort of nutritional firepower I needed to mount a counter offensive against cancer.

Kyo-Green is made by blending the best from land and sea—the concentrated juices of organically grown young barley leaves and wheat grass with kelp (a kind of seaweed), brown rice, and Bulgarian chlorella (a kind of algae).

Barley leaves and wheat grass are wonderful natural sources of vitamins and minerals—in particular vitamin A and beta carotene, excellent cancer fighting warriors—plus calcium, magnesium, and potassium. They are also rich in chlorophyll, great for cleaning and building the blood, plus detoxifying the liver, an essential part of my cancer battle plan. The brown rice in Kyo-Green works together with the barley leaves and wheat grass to provide complex carbohydrates for energy, while the kelp is an additional source of vital minerals.

The chlorella in green drinks, like the barley and wheat grass, is packed with chlorophyll. In fact, chlorella contains the highest concentration of chlorophyll of any known plant. It is also 50 to 60 percent protein, contains all eight essential amino acids, helps to balance the pH level of the blood, aid digestion, and stimulates the immune system. To say it has value to human health is an understatement.

There are several different sources of this treasured algae. Kyo-Green uses chlorella that is grown in the Black

Sea region of Bulgaria in water from natural hot springs. Professor Shigetoh Miyachi from the University of Tokyo, regarded as the world's leading authority on chlorella, has said this about Bulgarian chlorella:

- The growing environment and the growing method are the best and most natural.
- The composition of ingredients are superior.
- The digestibility is of the highest level.[10]

Kyo-Green is indeed a powerhouse against illness and disease! It became a vital soldier in my counter attack on cancer.

Garlic

The use of garlic for medicinal purposes can be traced back over 4,000 years to the ancient Egyptians. Modern-day scientists have been conducting studies with this condiment in an effort to see if folklore could be replaced with hard facts. No doubt to the amazement of some, studies have revealed that the 200 or so different compounds found in garlic have biological activities that can favorably influence the course of many diseases.

In the September 4, 1990 edition of the *New York Times,* nutrition writer Jane Brody noted that test results from various laboratory studies show that the ingredients in garlic are able to do the following:

- Suppress cholesterol synthesis by the liver, lowering total serum cholesterol by reducing only the harmful LDL cholesterol and leaving the protective HDL cholesterol at normal levels.
- Lower levels of triglycerides, another blood fat that has been linked to an increased risk of heart attacks.
- Reduce the tendency of the blood to clot, more

effectively even than aspirin, and help the body dissolve existing clots, effects that may ward off heart attacks and strokes.

◆ Promote regression of fatty deposits in blood vessels and perhaps reverse arterial blockages caused by atherosclerosis.

◆ Block the ability of chemical carcinogens to transform normal cells into cancer cells and in some cases inhibit the early growth of trans- formed cells.

◆ Stimulate various immunological factors that may help the body combat cancer as well as stubborn fungal infections, like Candida albicans, a yeast that plagues millions.

◆ Protect cells against damage by oxidizing agents and heavy metals that are wide spread in modern industrial environments.[11]

At the recommendation of my nutritionist, I added garlic to my cancer battle plan. But not just any garlic would do. She favored an odorless, aged garlic extract called KYOLIC, made by the same folks who make Kyo-Green.

KYOLIC is the only aged garlic extract made from garlic grown in organically pure soil—free of pesticides, fungicides, pherbicides, and other chemical contaminants. In order to preserve all of the garlic's important sulfur compounds, vitamins, minerals, enzymes, and amino acids, a unique twenty-month natural cold-aging process is employed.

No other garlic supplement has received the recognition that KYOLIC has. In fact, at a symposium I attended where 500 medical doctors and scientists came together to discuss nutrition in the treatment of cancer, KYOLIC was the only commercial product allowed to be represented. Dr. Willem H. Khoe, M.D., Ph.D., observed, "The use of garlic, and especially KYOLIC, has been a great improvement in the care of what I call the diseases of modern civilization."[12]

Dr. Liu (Pennsylvania State University) revealed that nitrosamines are the most common cancers in the world and are caused by the air we breathe, the food we eat, and the water we drink. His testing showed that KYOLIC proved to be more effective than even vitamin C against these carcinogens.

Desiccated Liver

"Glandular or organo-therapy is based on the premise that *like cells help like cells.*"[13] For this reason I supplemented my live foods diet with desiccated liver in an attempt to lend a helping hand to my own liver. It works synergistically with B-complex vitamins to heal and restore damaged livers, clean and build the blood, and restore the acid-alkaline balance. My "chemotherapy-wounded" liver and blood were thankful for the help.

Author Marjorie Holmes' explanation is appropriate: Desiccated liver "is simply raw liver from which fat and fiber have been removed. It is then vacuum-dried in a low-heat process that doesn't destroy its precious nutrients. In fact, a mere teaspoon of desiccated liver packs more concentrated iron and vitamin B than a whole pound of cooked liver. . . . [It] is not only a terrific energizer, it can help detoxify the poisons that now assault us from almost everything we eat, touch or even breathe."[14]

Pancreatic Enzymes

As with the desiccated liver, pancreatic enzymes were also taken in light of the help my liver needed. Pancreatic enzymes are normally activated by the liver and are important to food digestion. By supplying my body with an outside source of these enzymes, good digestion was assured to keep precious nutrients flowing to promote healthy cell life. In other words, by taking these enzyme tablets with my meals, a load was taken off my liver so it had a chance to heal. These enzymes are also known to attack the coating on cancer cells, exposing them to the immune system for destruction.

SUMMARY

Dr. Harold W. Harper has written, "Degenerative diseases are not caused by viruses, bacteria, or parasites, but by the body's inadequate metabolic response to a condition in which the cells of the body are being slowly poisoned by too many of the wrong things or not enough of the right things at the right time."[15]

Calling in dietary reinforcements is an effort to help supply the body with the "right things" that it is lacking in order to provide optimum health. Consult with your nutritionist to see exactly which vitamins, minerals, and miscellaneous nutrients may be lacking in your body. It is up to the body to take these nutrients and build healthy cells. There are no guarantees that it will. Supplementation, however, provides the body with an opportunity. In my case, it was very helpful.

CHAPTER
VI

Principle Five—
Maintain Morale

D uring the war in the Persian Gulf, the world watched as the United States and its allies put to flight the Iraqi army that had invaded the country of Kuwait. It was an amazingly swift victory for the allies, for much had been made in the press of the Iraqi resolve to make this "the mother of all battles."

Under commanding General "Stormin'" Norman Schwarzkopf's watchful eye, the battle plan had been designed to use all available forces to come at the Iraqis in unrelenting fashion. The enemy was engaged in the air, on land, and at sea. This was a war the allies were not going to lose!

In the end, the major factor contributing to the demise of the massive Iraqi force was its lack of troop morale. They'd simply lost the will to fight. At every opportunity, thousands were surrendering--laying down their arms and giving up. A war that some people had predicted would last for quite some time came to an early end.

Within this history of recent warfare there is an

107

important lesson for those of us battling cancer. *Only those who have determined in their minds to fight have any chance to win.* Your battle with cancer is as much mental as it is physical. It begins with an inner commitment to wage war.

In his book entitled *Anatomy of an Illness*, Norman Cousins tells the story of how he successfully overcame a crippling disease that threatened to take him to an early grave:

> People have asked me what I thought when I was told by the specialists that my disease was progressive and incurable. The answer is simple. Since I didn't accept the verdict, I wasn't trapped in the cycle of fear, depression, and panic that frequently accompanies a supposedly incurable illness. I must not make it seem, however, that I was unmindful of the seriousness of the problem or that I was in a festive mood throughout. Being unable to move my body was all the evidence I needed that the specialists were dealing with real concerns. But deep down, I knew I had a good chance and relished the idea of bucking the odds.[1]

Cousins' example is just one of many in which people just like you and me have dealt successfully with life-threatening diseases and gloomy diagnoses by first determining in their minds that they were going to put up a fight. My files and bookshelves are filled with such stories.

A newspaper clipping came into my possession not long ago about a woman who had gone head to head with a bad case of breast cancer. Seems she'd talked her surgeons into letting her watch a video replay of her double mastectomy. "When I saw the size of the tumor, I knew what I was up against," she said. "It was not a vagrant cell. It was a formidable enemy I knew would kill me."[2]

During her recovery period in the hospital she'd pored over all the cancer studies available to her in the hospital's library. In the process, she discovered two very interesting things. First, in Japan, China, Thailand, and the Philippines low rates of breast cancer were being linked to a low fat diet. Second, several studies had linked the growth of cancerous cells with a lack of oxygen transference in the blood system.

Armed with information and hope, she steeled her resolve to fight. Vegetarian became her diet (no meat, fish, or dairy products); exercise became her passion. "I started feeling great and regaining control over my life," she says. That was eight years ago. No trace of cancer today. She's winning the war because she decided to fight.

Health and healing, fighting disease and winning— these are not just issues of body mechanics and medical technology. The spirit of the person must also be engaged—the mind, the emotions, the will to live.

In recent years Bernie Siegel, M.D., has become well-known among cancer fighters for his book *Love, Medicine and Miracles.* His primary thesis is that the cancer patient stands a much better chance of overcoming the disease if he or she enters the ring emotionally ready to take the fight right to the opponent. He notes that a group of research scientists in London "recently reported a ten-year survival rate of 75% among cancer patients who reacted to the diagnosis with a 'fighting spirit', compared with a 22% survival rate among those who responded with 'stoic acceptance' or feelings of helplessness or hopelessness."[3]

There is, indeed, a strong link between mind and body; an obvious bond between the spirit of a man and his health. Hippocrates recognized this thousands of years ago. He is known to have respected the importance of helping the patient by reaching the mind as well as dealing with the body. King Solomon of ancient Israel, considered by many to have been the wisest man who ever lived, revealed a similar understanding of the mind-body link in his writings. He observed, "A man's spirit sustains him in sickness, but a crushed spirit who can bear?"

Not only do our minds and emotions play an important role in fighting cancer once we have it, there is also evidence that our mind-set can play a role in our getting cancer in the first place. A wealth of scientific studies reveal that chronic stress and negative emotions (worry, fear, anxiety, bitterness, anger, etc.) can cause hormonal and chemical imbalances in the body resulting in a metabolism that is fertile ground for the development of cancer. "The British Medical Association states that there is not a single cell of the body that is totally removed from the influence of mind and emotions."[4]

Today experts such as Dr. Bernie Siegel, Norman Cousins, and many others are helping restore to the high-tech world of modern medicine the long-held understanding that, in each of us, a strong "mind-body" link affects our health significantly. We're learning that we need to take our emotional temperature each day, being willing to deal quickly with toxic emotions and negative stresses that may have a long-term poisonous impact on our metabolic systems if we allow them to ferment and fester. That would be like sabotage in our war on cancer.

The fact that you already have cancer makes the importance of developing an emotional climate that is conducive to fighting it even more imperative. The enemy has broken through your defenses. It's going to take serious combat to push it back.

In my own combat with cancer, the following attitudes have helped me to keep my spirit detoxified and properly fed.

◆ Taking charge
◆ Refusing to play victim
◆ Saying no to slavery
◆ Practicing thankfulness
◆ Finding humor
◆ Setting goals

TAKING CHARGE

Odd as it may seem, even when faced with death, the fear of failure keeps some people from taking charge of their personal war on cancer.

Dr. Siegel observed that "60-70% [of cancer patients] are like actors auditioning for a part. They perform to satisfy the physician. They act the way they think the doctor wants them to act, hoping that then the doctor will do all the work and the medicine won't taste bad. They'll take their pills faithfully and show up for appointments. They'll do what they're told—unless the doctor suggests radical changes in their lifestyle—but it never occurs to them to question the doctor's decisions or strike out on their own by doing things for themselves that just 'feel right'. These are the people who, given a choice, would rather be operated on than actively work to get well."[5]

I know those feelings. For a time following my diagnosis, I struggled with whether or not I really wanted to fight for my life. My prognosis was bleak. I didn't know if anyone else had been healed from cancer as far spread as mine. Was fighting even worth it? Sure, I'd agreed to follow through with all the treatments my oncologist ordered. But that wouldn't be fighting. That would be playing it safe. That would be having things done *to* me, not *by* me. If the treatments failed and I died, it wouldn't be me who was the failure. It'd be the oncologist. Or it'd be the inadequacies of those cancer-fighting therapies. But it wouldn't be me. In effect, I wanted to hide behind my doctor.

However, he'd already told me the truth of the limitations of what he could do for me. He'd already told me that the chemotherapy would only work for a while before the cancer would become resistant. He'd already predicted that I'd be dead within two years under the types of therapy he could offer. He'd already said, "Anne, I can't cure you, but maybe I can help keep you alive long enough for you to learn how to cure yourself."

It was clear that if I was to survive, I was going to have to work hard toward health and healing. I was going to have to go beyond the limitations of what medicine had to offer. But as I said, I was struggling with the fear of failure. This was, after all, stage four cancer. The worst! What if I gave it my best shot and came up short? During my whole life I'd grown accustomed to doing less than my best for fear that if I did my very best it would not be good enough.

My husband helped me to see things in a new light. "Your body is like a garden God has given you to take care of," he said. "Right now, it's full of weeds. Your job, until He reclaims the garden, is to do your best at getting rid of the weeds and growing the good stuff. Failure is not found in giving the garden back (dying)—that's going to happen to all of us sooner or later—but in doing less than your best with it while it's yours."

His simple illustration helped me clarify my role in the war being waged for my body. My fear of failure was replaced by a sense of responsibility, a sense of stewardship. As long as I had the body, the responsibility of working for its health was mine.

❖   ❖   ❖

POINTS TO PONDER

Good health does not come easily; you must work for it.
—Charles B. Simone, M.D.,
Cancer and Nutrition

*The question we must answer is do we really want
to take charge of ourselves. . . . When I was in practice
in Plymouth, it was quite common for me to have to say
to a patient, "Look—if you don't change your eating
habits or way of life, you'll always be ill with
this particular problem and will have to take drugs
to keep you comfortable for the rest of your life."
Generally, after a short pause for thought,
the answer was, "Give me the pills."*

—Alec Forbes, M.D.,
The Famous Bristol Detox Diet for Cancer Patients

❖　　❖　　❖

REFUSING TO PLAY VICTIM

If you're going to have any chance of beating cancer, you
must enter the fight with the attitude that you'll do everything possible to win—that you will be its victor, not its
victim. *Playing the role of victim is the most destructive
attitude a person with cancer can entertain.* Those who do
tend toward passive acceptance of what they've been told
is their inevitable fate. They tend to fulfill the prophecies
made of them, dying right on schedule, in line with their
prognosis. The term *victim* suggests that others should
feel sorry for them, take care of them, make their decisions for them.

On the other hand, there are those individuals who,
no matter what their prognosis may be, refuse to be
labeled as victims. Dr. Siegel refers to these as "excep-
tional patients," observing that 15 to 20 percent of cancer
patients fit this description. "They educate themselves
and become specialists in their own care. They question the doctor because they want to understand their
treatment and participate in it. They demand dignity,
personhood, and control, no matter what the course of
the disease."[6]

If you're going to beat this disease effectively, you must not play the role of passive victim. If you do, cancer will have its way with you. It will take what you give, and keep taking, until finally there is nothing else of you to take.

As part of the therapy program, my oncologist had T-shirts made for his cancer patients with the logo "Kick Cancer's Butt." Three times a week we gathered at the local health club to ride the lifecycles and pump iron. No "victims" allowed, thank you. Just warriors! Another woman in the group commented, "This is the one thing I can do for myself that helps me feel like I'm taking control." She was still unaware of other things she could have been doing, but this was a start. She was beginning her journey away from feeling like the victim—toward becoming the victor.

Other professionals in the field of cancer treatment are recognizing the powerful effects of exercise in helping people put aside feelings of being a victim. The Simontons, mentioned in chapter 4, wrote,

> Several studies have observed that people on regular exercise programs (specifically, a combination of walking and jogging) tend to be more flexible in their thinking and beliefs, they tend to have an increased sense of self-sufficiency, a strengthened self-concept, improved self-acceptance, less tendency to blame others, and less depression. The overall picture is that people engaged in regular exercise programs tend to develop a healthier psychological profile in general—one often identified with a favorable prognosis for the course of the malignancy.[7]

SAYING NO TO SLAVERY

I remember in high school in the late sixties being shown a film about the dangers of smoking. The key figure in the film had undergone surgery to remove cancerous tumors from his mouth and throat. He'd also had a tube put in just above his breastbone, through which he breathed. It was not a pretty sight! But one moment in the film has stayed with me all these years: that man stuck a lit cigarette into the tube in his chest to take a drag. He knew it was killing him, but he kept right on doing it. Smoking had ruined his health, yet he continued to allow it to have control over his life.

The National Cancer Institute has been telling us for years that smoking can and does cause cancer. Of the 460,000 or so people who die in the U.S. each year because of cancer, roughly 30 percent contract the disease because of smoking. This year and next year, and no doubt for years to come, nearly 140,000 people are going to forfeit their lives simply because they refuse to quit putting burning leaves to their lips (or chest tubes, as the case may be).

Next to smoking, diet causes more cancer in the U.S. than anything else. "Diet is the #2 killer of Americans," observed Dr. Michael McGinnis, director of the office of disease prevention and health promotion at the U.S. Department of Health and Human Services.[8] It, too, can be enslaving. I was recently talking with a cancer cousin after he'd seen his nutritionist. "I found out that my diet is feeding my cancer," he said, "but I don't know if life would be worth living if I have to give up steak."

I have observed that because we tend to become emotionally enslaved to the foods we eat, many people with cancer would rather continue to have nasty things done to them than to make decided changes in their eating habits. We more readily subject our bodies to cutting, burning, and poisoning (surgery, radiation, chemotherapy) than do something really "radical" and horrible like (*gulp*) choosing to eat differently.

Forced into the nutritional therapy as my last possible

hope, I discovered that life is still good, even if I can't eat the foods I used to eat. I also made the amazing discovery that tastes can and do change. Each day now, when I consistently do what I know is right and good for my physical health via my diet, my emotional well-being is enhanced. A cycle of encouragement is formed. Doing right for my body helps my morale. Good morale helps my body do more effective battle against the possible return of cancer.

PRACTICING THANKFULNESS

Thankfulness is not an easy attitude to develop, especially when you're locked in mortal battle for your life. It's even harder when there's anger involved at others who have seemingly played a role in your troubles. I was very upset with the family doctor who misdiagnosed my cancer for a year. I was angry at the emergency room doctor who seemed to think my pain was all in my head. I was angry at the mammography doctor who, way back in the beginning, had assured me in no uncertain terms that my lumps were not cancerous.

I had a lot to be angry about. To have left my anger unattended would have allowed it to fester and ferment, rotting away at my ability to focus effectively on regaining my health. Anger is like a cancer of the mind, devouring the emotional energies of a person. Just like my body, my mind and spirit needed detoxification. All the emotional poisons in my head needed to be cleaned out before my body could effectively work toward healing.

So I dealt with my anger in a way that worked for me. I got it all out on paper. I've been keeping a journal for years. Journaling then became my way of identifying and letting go of my damaging emotions. First I wrote letters to all the doctors who had treated me so poorly. I actually mailed a copy of one of these angry letters to my family physician to let him know how much he had let me down.

Then I wrote letters to God, venting my anger and disappointment at Him for allowing all this terrible stuff to happen to me. Since high school I have felt that God is knowable in a personal way. I made His acquaintance as the result of a project aimed at discovering the foundational truth about life. My quest had taken me to the Bible, where I discovered the love of God enfleshed in a man named Jesus, who claimed to be God's Son. But now I was angry at God for all that had happened. He could have protected me, but He hadn't. I knew that I didn't want to be angry at Him for long, because I loved Him. But I also knew that it was important for me to get my feelings out in the open.

For me, it was therapeutic to have gone through this process of untangling the reasons for my anger. I saw the specific issues underlying my strong emotions and dealt with them in specific ways. For instance, I realized that God had not caused my cancer or wished it on me, but in the laws of nature had allowed it. As sure as "what goes up must come down" and "cows don't fly," diet impacts health. The biblical principle that "a man reaps what he sows" applies to health and diet as much as it does to anything else in life. The phrase "you are what you eat" is true. God is all-powerful and could have protected me from developing a diet-related degenerative disease, but He seldom breaks the natural laws He has set in place to govern His creation.

I suppose I could have continued to be angry at God for not making me an exception to His rules, but I began to see my own responsibility in this whole mess. And yes, some of the doctors I was forced to deal with had been inadequate in their treatment of me. But hey, doctors aren't perfect. Just like car mechanics, body mechanics sometimes make mistakes. It was important for me emotionally, physically, and spiritually to come to a point where I could honestly say I had forgiven them in my heart. This was hard, but it needed to be done for my own well-being. It helped to read the Bible and be reminded of all that my Creator had forgiven me.

As I worked to rid my spirit of the emotional poisons of anger, there was yet another hurdle in my path before giving thanks could become a full-fledged member of my war cabinet. It had to do with an attitude of feeling sorry for myself, of feeling like I'd been cheated or robbed of what was supposed to be mine in life. I'd lost a breast and a great deal of my self-esteem as a woman. My hair was gone because of the chemotherapy, and I was forced into the indignity of having a fifteen-inch tube hanging from my chest, like I was some sort of robo-patient. It just wasn't fair.

Then one day, early in my war, I read a magazine article about a man who had undergone surgery to remove his nose, which had become cancerous. A picture of his tortured and misshapen face was included. His sad story reminded me that no matter how bad my own situation was, someone else would always seem to have things worse. Perhaps not the noblest of motivations, but it worked for me.

From that day on I've made it a daily routine to make lists in my journal of all the things I have to thank God for. It's amazing what this has done for my spirit—and in turn for my body. When I find myself bemoaning my losses or feeling sorry for myself, I'm often reminded of the man with no nose. I hope that he too has found a way of turning his spirit toward thankfulness.

Here is one entry I made in my journal shortly after my commitment to give thanks:

> While sitting in our family doctor's office the other day, I saw a woman come in with a young boy. She was quite obviously a burn victim. I could see that parts of her face, neck, chest, and arms were

disfigured. The thing that radiated from this person was anger. Everything in the way she walked, talked, slammed doors, and treated people said, "I am a victim. I'm mad as hell, and everybody around me is going to suffer because of it."

This had a profound effect on me. First of all, I realized that we choose our attitudes, the kind of person we are going to be, in spite of our circumstances. This woman chose anger and tried to punish those around her. I choose love and acceptance, and even joy and peace. My source is God and a life I surrendered to Him twenty years ago. I choose to be a channel of comfort to those around me.

Second, it reminded me that I have a lot to be thankful for. Yes, I will have some ugliness and disfigurement on my road—but there are others who have it worse than I do. I have so much to be thankful for. The point is, I am choosing that what radiates from me will be genuine thankfulness. Every day I will count my blessings in order to emphasize what I have been given, not what has been taken away.

❖ ❖ ❖

POINT TO PONDER

To ignore God at any time in one's life
is a foolishness I find difficult to understand;
to ignore Him while staring sickness and disease
in the face is more than foolish.
—Dr. Richard O. Brennan,
Coronary? Cancer? God's Answer: Prevent It!

❖ ❖ ❖

FINDING HUMOR

I found this quote in a book I have at home: "Medical experts tell us laughter is healthy. In fact, it is bad to suppress laughter. It goes back down and spreads your hips. Imagine how painful it would be if it settled in your colon."9

A picture comes to mind of a person bent over in agony, his arms wrapped tightly around his middle. His bowels are rumbling with the echoes of riotous laughter that have become stuck down there. His face is puffed and twisted, red with pain. One is left to wonder what laughter feels and sounds like when released from the inappropriate end. Or what would happen if this guy were rushed to the hospital for surgery? Would peals of laughter escape with a "whoosh" when the incision was made?

Funny thoughts, right? Funny thoughts are important. They helped me wage successful war on my cancer.

A morphine-like substance secreted by the human brain, called endorphin, acts as a natural anesthesia and relaxant. When it enters the bloodstream, a person experiences a heightened sense of well-being. It is possible that laughter stimulates the release of endorphin. Humor has a way of washing away the emotional toxins from the mind, lifting the spirit, and providing new perspective to life's problems. King Solomon also wrote, "A cheerful heart does good like medicine, but a broken spirit makes a person sick."

In an effort to add laughter to my cancer-fighting arsenal, I began to look for humor wherever I could find it. I used my journal to record the bits of humor in my unfortunate circumstances. For instance, it occurred to me that being bald wasn't so bad after all. Think of all the money I was saving on shampoo and haircuts.

In some cases I tried to create humor. My mother, sister, and I turned my hunt for a suitable wig into a wonderfully funny experience—and long-term memory. We took a camera with us to a local wig boutique and captured how we each looked in everything from a "Cher" to a "Dr. Ruth."

I also made it a point to import humor from the world around me. I watched funny movies, read the comics in the newspaper (especially *Calvin and Hobbes*), watched funny shows on television, and listened to Rush Limbaugh on the radio. With the help of my family, I sought to create an environment of humor and lightheartedness that would counteract the negative effects and emotions of cancer. Nothing like belly laughs to relieve stress and begin to change body chemistry.

Norman Cousins wrote,

> Some people, in the grip of uncontrollable laughter, say their ribs are hurting. The expression is probably accurate, but it is delightful "hurt" that leaves the individual relaxed almost to the point of an open sprawl. It is the kind of "pain," too, that most people would do well to experience every day of their lives. It is as specific and tangible as any other form of physical exercise. Though its biochemical manifestations have yet to be as explicitly charted and understood as the effects of fear or frustration or rage, they are real enough.[10]

SETTING GOALS (DREAM THERAPY)

When we were first told that my time was probably short, our lives came to a screeching halt. Life stood still as we tried to figure out how people manage to carry on daily existence with the guarantee of impending doom hanging over their heads. Everything about our lives had become so heavy, so overwhelming—and at the same time our resolve to carry on had become so limp.

The turning point came when we decided to set goals to shoot for with whatever time I had left. My husband called it "dream therapy." Together we identified things we'd always wanted to do or accomplish, but had put off for "someday." Suddenly, "someday" was upon us. The curse of cancer had given us license to put other less important things aside and move more directly toward our heartfelt goals.

One of the most encouraging and emotionally rewarding things I did was to start my own business. Ever since childhood, when I sat for hours at a time with pad and pencil designing dream homes, I'd wanted to be an interior decorator. With the printing of brochures and business cards, "Anne Elizabeth Decorating" was launched. I didn't make a lot of money, but that wasn't the point. Accomplishing the lifelong dream of starting my own interior decorating business paid emotional dividends that money could never have purchased. I got just enough jobs to keep my spirit continually supplied with cancer-fighting nutrients, while not overly taxing my physical strength. I was bringing beauty into my world, which in turn was helping to bring health into my body.

It's amazing how being given the cancer "death sentence" actually accelerated real living for me—and for our whole family. Things that we'd always wanted to do became reality because we made them a priority. We'd always wanted to do more memory building activities with our two kids, yet we never seemed to find time until cancer forced us to make time. Once we'd determined that memory making was one of our goals, we bought a twenty-year-old recreational vehicle (which affectionately became known as Charlie Brown). What fun we had in that old hunk of junk! Again, more emotional nutrients for my spirit.

During my stay in the hospital when I was first diagnosed with cancer, friends brought by the usual array of flowers, cards, and plants to decorate my room and brighten my spirit. Often gifts of this sort serve a short-term purpose and are discarded. The flowers fade, the plants die, and most cards, after one more reading, are tossed. However, in this case, one small plant survived and is still with us today, several years later. Repotted and much larger, it now sits in a prominent place in our home where it reminds us daily how important it is to keep watering our dreams.

I'll never forget the day I came home from the hospital. In the mailbox a letter awaited me. Opening the envelope, I found an invitation. As I read it, tears trickled down my face. There on a folded piece of notebook paper, printed neatly in crayon, was an invitation to my daughter Jessica's wedding. At the space for an RSVP were these words: "Please be there." She was only ten years old—here were words to live for. I had a wedding to attend.

The process of dreaming dreams and setting goals kept me moving forward with eager anticipation into my future. There's something life giving about that, a regeneration of the spirit within. After a time, every single dream and goal I'd originally written down had been accomplished. Even the ones I'd considered impossible had been achieved. So I came up with new dreams and goals. This book is part of that continuing list, as is our vision for HealthQuarters. I mentioned at the end of chapter 1 that my husband and I have begun an organization aimed at serving the information, education, and encouragement needs of fellow cancer cousins. We're not entirely sure of all that lies ahead, but we're looking forward with eager anticipation to the adventure of moving toward our dreams.

How about you? What are your dreams, your goals, the things you've always wanted to do or accomplish that you've been putting off for "someday"? Again from wise King Solomon comes an important insight about life: "Hope delayed makes the heart sick, but when dreams finally come true, there is life and joy."

FIELDING YOUR DREAMS
I have always wanted to . . .

_____

_____

_____

_____

_____

_____

_____

_____

_____

_____

_____

_____

Just as our bodies need daily exercise, so do our attitudes. The following worksheet is designed to help develop emotional health and strength in the continuing war on cancer. You may want to answer these questions daily in your own journal.

DAILY ATTITUDE WORKOUT

- ◆ What can I do to take charge of my fight for health today?

- ◆ Will I play the part of cancer victim or victor today?

- ◆ Are there changes I need to make today to help my body fight?

- ◆ What things can I thank God for today?

- ◆ How could I bring humor into my life today?

- ◆ How can I move toward my dreams and goals today?

VII

Principle Six— Carefully Select Your Professional Help

Not long ago I received a phone call from a woman who had read a story in the local newspaper about my successful battle against cancer. She was a cancer warrior herself, in need of encouragement.

"How do you find a doctor who really wants to help you?" she asked, desperation sounding through her voice.

As she reviewed the details of her story with me, desperation turned to anger. Seems she'd become concerned about two lumps she'd found in her breast during a self-examination. A mammogram suggested that they were not cancerous, but she remained unconvinced.

"I went to five different doctors before one would agree to do a biopsy on me," she sobbed into the phone. "Finally this one jerk of a doctor agreed to do it, but he treated me like I was a complete idiot. He said, 'Okay, okay, we'll just do it. It'll take three minutes, and I'll come right back and show you that it's just a cyst,'" she continued. "When he did come back into the room, he was all embarrassed because it was cancerous. Then he did the larger lump and found it was cancerous, too.

"I felt like hitting him!" she admitted. "Not because of the cancer, but because he'd treated me like I was just a silly woman, worried about nothing and wasting his time."

I told her that I was proud of her. She had accomplished rule number one in the process of forming a team of professionals to help her win her war. That rule is "take command." She had met resistance, but had pressed to get the information she needed.

In the war against cancer, you're the general. It's your body, your health, your money. Everyone else is hired help. Their role is to assist you to accomplish your goal of health and healing by lending their specialized expertise to the project. Just like the woman I spoke to on the phone, it's entirely possible that in your own battle for health, you're going to be emotionally abused by the very people to whom you've turned for help—health professionals, some of whom present themselves as insensitive and arrogant. Don't give up. Don't allow the hired help to take command while you play the role of passive bystander. Your life may depend on it!

But the caller's question remains to be answered. How do you find health professionals who *really* want to be helpful? To that query I will add another. What kinds of health fields need to be represented on your team?

FIELDS AND PHILOSOPHIES
My own experience has been that I've needed an oncologist, a nutritionist, a metabolic physician, and a chiropractor on my war cabinet. Together they have provided me with a full spectrum of information necessary to be aware of my options and opportunities to treat my disease.

Oncologist
Oncologists know the facts about chemotherapy. They are also your link to surgery and radiation therapy. This

doesn't mean I'm recommending their therapies. That's a choice that only you can make. It is important, though, to have an oncologist on your team in case you decide to go with one of the "big three."

Oncologists are also equipped to keep track of the rate of cancerous activity in your system. Although I am now fully committed to battling my cancer through metabolic therapy (nutrition), I continue to have lab work done by my oncologist to track my cancer count. I highly value his input on my progress. We have what I consider an excellent working relationship.

Regarding his philosophy, it takes a special kind of oncologist to continue seeing me when I've gone an entirely different direction in my therapy. Of course, when I actually made the switch to nutrition he had already said there was nothing more he could offer me within his field. That, no doubt, made it easier for him to accept my new direction. And yet, a couple of statements he has made at various times in our working relationship characterize the type of thinking you will want to look for in an oncologist should you decide to add one to your own team.

The first statement was previously mentioned in this book, but merits a repeat. "Anne," he said, "I can't cure you with chemotherapy, but perhaps I can keep you alive long enough for you to learn how to cure yourself." I liked that. This honest, humble statement showed that he knew the boundaries of what he could do for me. As promised, chemotherapy may have prolonged my life, but it didn't cure my disease. His honesty helped me realize early that I couldn't sit passively by and wait for chemotherapy to do something for me that he never promised it could. I would have to go beyond what he could offer.

A second statement that characterizes the philosophy you should watch for was made when it was obvious that my oncologist had been wrong in telling me that nutritional therapy would do me no good. "Well," he said, "I don't understand it, but I'm not one to argue with results." Some medical professionals are angry if you get well any way but their way. If you want to add an oncologist to your team, look for one who is willing to put your health and healing above the politics of how it happened. At the same time you must remember, he is an oncologist. He is trained to fight cancer with chemo. Don't expect or demand that he know much about nutritional therapy. If you want him to be honest about his boundaries, don't expect him to operate beyond them.

Nutritionist
When I first began to pursue nutrition as a cancer-fighting option, I shopped around for the right nutritionist. When I finally settled on one, I was amazed at the time she took to know my story and figure out what was going on in my body. I brought her a copy of an exhaustive blood test done at a local medical clinic, and she spent hours designing a plan of nutritional therapy that would meet my specific healing needs. This was not some pre-designed program straight from a book, but a tailor-made system of cleansing and rebuilding.

A common mistake is to consider nutritionists and dieticians as one and the same. They are not. My own experience with dieticians has been that many are concerned mainly with putting together a "balanced diet" (whatever that means) based on the principles of the four basic food groups. Their "service" to the cancer patient is to ensure that they keep weight on, especially as it relates to maintaining an appetite during chemotherapy treatments.

Early in my cancer fight, I attended a meeting for cancer patients at which the head dietician from a local hospital was the featured speaker. Knowing only a little about nutrition at that point, I was nonetheless shocked by what she was recommending that we put into our bodies. A lot of fatty, sugary, low fiber food—all consumed in an effort to keep the pounds on during chemotherapy. Ironic that the food she was recommending was the same kind linked to degenerative disease in the first place. Does that make sense to you? Me neither!

I complained to my oncologist about the stupidity of such nutritional nonsense. We got to talking about a common philosophy behind hospital food. While the cancer patient should be eating salad and drinking carrot juice to stimulate the immune system and liver functions, many dieticians offer fried chicken, mashed potatoes, chocolate chip cookies, and a soft drink. "Comfort food," my oncologist called it. "People who are fighting for their lives aren't very willing to change their diets."

"Maybe they would," I countered, "if someone in that hospital told them that diet was a major factor in the development of their disease."

Richard Brennan, M.D., makes an interesting point: "What a world of good the nurses could accomplish if they were better informed about the nutritional way to combat disease."[1] We can hope that, as Americans realize the common sense behind nutrition, one day such a thing will be confirmed. In the meantime, the current philosophy of many hospital staffs contains little if any understanding of nutritional therapy against cancer.

Nutritionists, on the other hand, are concerned with figuring out the specific foods that we need to eat to reestablish and maintain the health and vitality of the metabolic system. They are also concerned with detoxifying the body of toxic buildup so the nutrients in foods can be fully utilized. Discussions of juice fasting and bowel cleansing (enemas) are signals that you are in the presence of a true nutritionist.

Many nutritionists sell dietary supplements (vitamins, minerals, etc.). This makes all the sense in the world. They are, after all, the experts in this field. They know what products are on the market and which ones work the best. Why shouldn't they have these on hand for sale? The kind of nutritionist you want to find, however, is someone who is more concerned about counseling you than about selling you products. You'll be able to tell the difference.

Watch out for sales people who market themselves in the yellow pages as nutritional consultants. This doesn't mean that their products are bad, or that they have nothing of value to say. It's just that you need to know they may be more skilled in sales than in helping you with your unique nutritional needs.

I truly appreciate the nutritionist that God sent into my life. She's a unique person who cares deeply for the clients she advises. She's known for her innate wisdom in helping each person she works with—wisdom I believe comes from her personal relationship with God. I am of the opinion that the very best nutritionists are those who are able to see the bigger picture of life, just as she sees it, intimately designed by the hands of the Creator.

Metabolic Physician

A metabolic physician is a medical doctor who specializes in helping the body renew or maintain health through nutritional biochemistry. This type of doctor was initially trained in conventional medicine but has chosen to pursue additional training in the more traditional practices of preventive medicine and natural healing. He stands in the gap between the oncologist and the nutritionist, able to administer certain kinds of therapies that a nutritionist might recommend but can't legally render—therapies that an oncologist could legally render but doesn't normally make a part of his practice.

For me, one of those therapies was mega-doses of vitamin C administered intravenously. The medical literature presents a strong case for this kind of therapy against cancer. My nutritionist recommended it, but couldn't administer it. My oncologist could legally have administered it, but didn't practice it. My metabolic physician had both the willingness and the wherewithal.

"Dr. Sheets" is what my husband and I call him. That's not his name, but a reflection of the fact that he loves to give handouts. He's as much teacher as he is physician. For every sort of question we've posed, his verbal response has been accompanied with a wealth of written information from various medical resources to help us study and understand. If you're going to add a metabolic physician to your team, and probably you should, look for someone who is willing to take the time to help you learn.

Chiropractor

Because the body is a single unit, all of its systems must work together in harmony for optimum health to be achieved. The main objective of the specialist trained in the art of chiropractic is to ensure healthy functioning of the body's nervous system. This definition may clarify: "Chiropractic is a system of treatment of human diseases and injuries based on the premise that the nerve system controls all other systems and all physiological functions in the body; that interference with the nerve control of these systems impairs their function and induces disease by rendering the body less resistant to infection or other causes."[2]

To accomplish their purposes, chiropractors manipulate various structures in the body, particularly the spine, to ensure that nerves and nerve impulses from the brain to various organs are not being pinched off by misalignment. Proper nerve function helps the body operate in a self-healing way. The human body has an ability not possessed by any machine: It can repair itself. Keeping the nervous system healthy helps the body maintain that ability.

I appreciated my chiropractor's specialized role in helping my body win back its health, not only through chiropractic but through his dedication to nutrition as well. He wasn't a "one-dimensional" professional, unable to see beyond the boundaries of his specialty.

SYNERGISM AND NETWORKING

Synergy describes the combined efforts of the parts that make up the whole of something. For instance, the muscles in the body work synergistically to perform the functions of life. The individual players on a football team work synergistically to score a touchdown. The potential of the whole is much greater than the potential of the parts in isolation.

Synergism in the war on cancer is the process of drawing on each field and specialist for those contributions that you deem necessary to form an effective battle plan. To do this you must recognize that each field has its boundaries, each specialist has limits. As the general at the center of the campaign, you must know which resources are at your disposal and be able to call them into action when needed.

One of the very best ways to discover health professionals for your team is through networking with other cancer warriors. Someone once said, "If you wish to know the true value of a physician's work, do not ask the physician; ask his patients." This applies to all health professionals. I make it a practice to recommend the members of my own team when people ask me who I'm seeing. I'm able to tell them the strengths and boundaries of each one, enabling them to make an informed decision as to whether or not to pursue an appointment. Tapping into the experiences and contacts of others who are fighting their own battle with cancer is a dynamite way to bring synergism to the battle front.

If you can't find other cancer warriors to network with, consider one or more of these ideas:

- ◆ Check the yellow pages under: health, homeopathy, natural medicine, naturopathic physician, nutrition, nutritionist.
- ◆ Contact a chiropractor. Their schooling includes some nutritional training, and they are often in touch with the sorts of professionals you're looking for.
- ◆ Contact a local health food store. People there are often knowledgeable about nutritionists and metabolic physicians. They may also have information about cancer support groups in your area.
- ◆ Contact a colonic therapist from the yellow pages. Here, too, is a health professional who often rubs shoulders with the kinds of professionals you may be looking for.
- ◆ Contact local churches. Church offices are often a good starting point for locating cancer support groups in the community.
- ◆ Check a library or bookstore for a copy of *Third Opinion* by John M. Fink. It contains a lengthy section listing names and locations of cancer support groups.
- ◆ Contact the American Association of Naturopathic Physicians for a referral close to your area.
- ◆ Contact the American College of Advancement in Medicine (ACAM) for an M.D. or D.O. referral in your area. Ask about doctors who specialize in nutrition and/or can help you rebuild your immune function.

❖   ❖   ❖

POINTS TO PONDER

*Do not believe in an authority. Rather examine all that
an authority says. Put everything to the test. Let truth be
your authority, not authority your truth.*
—Joel Robbins, D.C.,
Health Through Nutrition

*No practitioner should be treated as the ultimate and
only authority on the subject of health care. Each can
offer you the benefit of what he or she has learned, but it
is up to you—using your common sense, instincts, past
experience, present needs, and future goals—to decide
whether what a practitioner concludes is true
and helpful to you. That is how you remain in charge.*
—Harvey and Marilyn Diamond,
Fit for Life II: Living Health

Nature makes the cure, the doctor's job is to aid nature.
—Hippocrates, "father of medicine"

*Find a doctor who believes God is greater than
the medical associations, and you have found a jewel.*
—Jason Winters,
Killing Cancer

VIII

Coming Alongside in the Battle

Perhaps you've been reading this book not because *you* have cancer but because you know someone who does. Perhaps you've suddenly found yourself drawn close to this war through an acquaintance or a friend. Or maybe cancer has come knocking unexpectedly at the door of your own home. Perhaps the disease has drafted a loved one into battle, and you're looking for ways you can help.

This chapter is dedicated to you, one of the "other soldiers" in the war on cancer. Let me applaud you for taking the time to read this book. And let me also say how important your role is in an overall cancer battle plan. Your attitude and responsiveness to your friend or family member have the potential to impact significantly how he or she fares in the war.

From my own war experiences, I have made several observations about how friends and family members can be of the most help and encouragement. I offer the following thoughts, hoping that you will find even more ways and means to come alongside effectively.

FAMILY: CREATE A TEAMWORK ENVIRONMENT

I once heard a man say to a doctor who was examining his sick wife, "Doc, whatever she's got, I've got." My immediate family (husband and two kids—then ages seven and ten) showed the same spirit of partnership and "oneness" to join the war with me. One of the most helpful things they did was to change their diets to match the one I needed to eat—a low fat, high fiber, raw foods diet. In other words, we worked together to change our family's food culture from the standard American diet (SAD) to a vegetarian diet. They ate the salads, juices, fruits, etc., that I was eating and gave up the meat, dairy products, eggs, and most of the other foods they'd been used to.

It wasn't easy. But once we all got on the same "bandwagon," it became a fun challenge and source of family unity. It would have been much more difficult to maintain the discipline I needed to change my diet if my family had not been willing to make the same changes with me. Their effort would have made the three musketeers proud—"All for one, and one for all." By the way, my family's health has improved markedly!

Reflecting his total commitment to teamwork, my husband went to every doctor's appointment with me, read several books on cancer, moved our entire family to another city when I went there for a summer's worth of treatment, and generally did everything he could to be by my side. Priorities were shifted, resources refocused, and lifestyles changed all for my sake. He made me feel like this was truly *our* battle, not just mine.

FRIENDS: STAY INVOLVED

Perhaps the single most important thing for a cancer warrior is to have a network of friends who will treat him or her as a living, breathing person with a future. I am living proof that cancer need not be considered an automatic death sentence. One of my best friends later admitted to me that during my lowest times—times when my future looked most doubtful—she purposely never called or visited. She was afraid of getting too close, of experiencing too much pain if I died. She was protecting herself. I can understand that. But such an attitude from a friend is devastating to the one in the throes of the battle.

Speaking from experience, cancer warriors need a constant diet of hope. Being excluded from intimate relationships by friends or family members sends a clear message that you're hopeless—that you're a "goner" so others are going to start living life without you. The continued involvement of friends is a great encouragement to the cancer warrior's efforts. Here are ways to stay involved.

Ask How the Cancer Patient Is Doing

When a person is dealing with a serious situation in life, he usually has a need to talk about it. I wanted and needed to have people ask me how I was doing and what I was feeling. I needed to vent. I needed to have people listen. I remember when an out-of-town guest was visiting in our home, not once did he ask how I was doing. I knew he cared, but he simply never asked. It was as if he thought the subject taboo, too painful for me to discuss openly. Or perhaps he was protecting himself from the awkwardness of not knowing what to say to me or how he could give me hope.

Rule of thumb: Asking conveys caring. Not asking conveys indifference, even if you don't mean it to. Don't be afraid to ask. You don't need to have correct responses, just the willingness to show you care. If by chance your friend would rather not talk about his battle at the moment, he'll let you know.

Practice Prayer

After asking about your friend's situation you will be better informed as to what to pray for him or her. If you're not one to pray, you may want to start for the benefit of your friend. To tell you the truth, some of my greatest times of encouragement came when people asked how I was doing, then took the time to pray for me on the spot. When I heard others doing business for me with God, it gave me a wonderfully satisfying sense of being taken care of, of being loved.

Rule of thumb: Ask! God is listening.

Lift the Load

When a person finds out that he or she has cancer, the details of daily living tend to take a back seat. In the face of a life-threatening disease, the motivation to keep the toilets scrubbed and the lawn mowed tends to wane. In my case, I was emotionally and physically unable to maintain the daily "homemaker" routine. I can't tell you how much I appreciated the helpers who periodically showed up at my door to do the things I couldn't. It was most helpful when they called ahead of time, suggested a time when they'd like to come over, and asked for a list of things to pick from that I needed to have done.

Bringing over a meal was an especially great way to meet a need during the weeks immediately following my mastectomy and hospitalization. We were grateful if the meal was packaged in disposable containers. It is a hassle for the family to keep track of which serving dish belongs to whom and figure out how to return them. It is also a good idea to ask about dietary concerns ahead of time.

Rule of thumb: Volunteer your help; don't wait to be asked. It's hard enough to need help; having to ask for it compounds the problem.

Send a Card

In keeping with the idea of staying involved, sending a card is a great idea. It tells your friend that she's being remembered.

Rule of thumb: Write a note that says you care. Don't let the poet do your work for you. A card without a personal note from you is like kissing your sister—all the parts are there, but the emotion is missing.

Send a Book

When I was first diagnosed with cancer, I was hungry for hope. I had to have it! I searched for and devoured any books I could find that told the stories of cancer survivors—men and women who had found a way to beat the disease. Such books became encouraging friends. I'd be pleased if you'd send a copy of this book to your friend or family member with cancer.

Send Money

If you're not in the habit of giving money to others in need, this would be a great time to develop the habit. The financial burden of fighting a degenerative disease like cancer can be crushing. Even with good insurance coverage, Dave and I still find ourselves trying to dig our way out from under a mound of debt due to uncovered medical bills and related costs. The emotional fallout of increasing financial pressures is counterproductive to the cancer-fighting process. One of the nicest things you can do for a friend with cancer is to send a check to help alleviate some of the financial burden.

Rule of thumb: Send what you would like to receive, if you found yourself in the same boat, according to your ability.

❖   ❖   ❖

POINT TO PONDER

The mental condition of the patient and psychological cooperation of the family and the environment play

important roles in the restoration of the body. Every
patient needs faith, love, hope and encouragement.
—Max Gerson, M.D.,
A Cancer Therapy

❖   ❖   ❖

SUPPORTING THE HELPER (THOUGHTS FROM DAVE)

The focus of this chapter has been on how you can come
alongside the cancer warrior to give help and encouragement in the battle. Let me turn the attention to the needs
of the spouse when cancer comes to a married couple.

As the spouse of a cancer warrior, I learned firsthand
the stresses and frustrations of being thrust into the role
of caretaker. It's a tough role to play. You are cast as the
"silent partner," the person behind the scenes charged
with keeping everything together and running smoothly.
While your spouse is getting most of the attention from
those concerned (and rightly so), you are often being run
ragged trying to keep up with increased responsibilities,
pressing demands, and a never-ending pile of bills. The
pressures of maintaining a "one man show," which was
once a team effort, can be overwhelming. All this is com-
pounded, of course, by the fear of losing your mate.

So how do you effectively help and encourage a friend
or family member who is taking care of a spouse with cancer? Based on my own experience, the following thoughts
come to mind.

Let the Helper Know that You Care

There are two hurting people when one spouse is seriously ill. Sometimes the healthy one gets overlooked, lost
in the shuffle. Letting that person know that you care and
are specifically praying for him or her lifts the spirit and
lightens the load.

When I first learned that my wife was "hopelessly" ill

with cancer, I felt very much alone. I'd go home from the hospital at night with a huge lump in my throat, wondering what life would be like without my partner at my side. I'd look around the house, imagining its future emptiness without the presence of my best friend. My heart would hurt for my kids, so young to face losing a mother, and the terrible loneliness they must be feeling.

Phone calls from extended family members and friends helped me feel like others knew my pain. They asked questions about how Anne was doing. They asked about how I was feeling and how they could help. I didn't always know what to say to them, but their calls let me know that they were with me in and through the crisis.

I especially appreciated hearing that people were praying for us. I remember one night in particular when I was with a group of friends and they prayed together specifically for me. I had been so overwhelmed by all that I had to deal with that when they asked what they could pray about, all I could do was weep. Hearing these friends pray made me realize, again, that I wasn't alone in the battle.

Find Out What Would Help the Most

When my wife came home from the hospital, it fell on my shoulders to be nurse and housekeeper, along with everything else I was responsible for in life. It would have been easy for others to make wrong assumptions about the sort of help I needed most. For instance, since I am a man, others could have easily assumed that I would enjoy having someone else clean house. Truth was, I loved to clean house, do dishes, and wash clothes. Doing those things made me feel like I had control over my circumstances. Including them in my daily caretaking routine gave me a sense of emotional balance in the face of an unstable situation. I would have preferred that someone invite my kids out for a swim or a fun movie or a trip to the zoo.

Each person in a helper's role is unique. Each helper's felt needs will be different. The help you want to offer may not match the real wants and desires of the person. It's important to take the initiative to ask what kinds of help he or she would really find most beneficial. Ask the person to make a list, a wish list, of the kinds of things he'd most appreciate having done. Have him update it weekly. In other words, give the list time boundaries. Each new week is an opportunity to make a new list based on the changing emotions and circumstances in the home.

If the help your friend needs is not something you are able to provide, perhaps you can be instrumental in finding someone else who can. In so doing, you may find yourself being helpful in a way you never considered.

Allow the Person the Freedom to Be Himself

Some contend that everyone has the universal need to talk about personal problems with others. Perhaps that's true. If it is, it must be true in degrees. I've met people with ailing spouses who needed and appreciated a great deal of interaction with others. As for me, I needed more time by myself to reflect and write out my thoughts in a journal. Thinking and writing is my way of sorting through my emotions. I sometimes resented people's well-meaning attempts to render encouragement by trying to fill my hours with their presence.

One couple, knowing this about me, made it a point to ask me if I was getting enough time alone to recharge my "batteries." They often made time in their own schedule to take on my responsibilities at home so I could get away and be by myself for a while. Their sensitivity to my individual needs and uniqueness was gratifying. It made me feel like my need for time alone was legitimate—not only legitimate, but necessary.

In the end, one principle should guide all attempts to be helpful to someone who is taking care of a seriously ill spouse: *individualized attention and involvement.* We all need to know that others are willing to take the initiative to become aware of what we are feeling and going through. We each need to know that others will initiate coming alongside to help in whatever way is truly desired.

❖   ❖   ❖

Cancer need not be a death knell for everyone involved. It can be the greatest battle toward *life* for the cancer patient and each person who loves him or her. May you join forces with courage and hope—and win the war!

A

C-Rations

Following are low fat, high fiber, live enzyme, high alkaline recipes for the cancer patient in the rebuilding and maintaining stage. All vegetables should be fresh, unless otherwise noted. You can adjust the quantities as needed, depending on the number of people you plan to feed.

❖   ❖   ❖

BAKED POTATO BAR
Bake potatoes to minimum doneness.

Serve combination of these chopped ingredients over potatoes:

black olives	broccoli
green onions	green peppers
mushrooms	tomatoes

If desired top with ranch dressing:
1/2 C. Nayonaise (brand name; add water to thin)
1 tsp. onion (grated)
1/2 tsp. Spike (brand name)

❖   ❖   ❖

BLTs
Bread—two slices of 100 percent wholewheat, toasted
Lettuce—green leaf
Tomato—firm, *not* overripe

Spread toast with Nayonaise and/or Dijon mustard.

Optional: Add a slice of avocado.

Note: Forget the popular iceberg lettuce. It's nutritionally useless, if not possibly harmful.

❖   ❖   ❖

Brown Rice Banzai

Cook whole grain brown rice, according to package directions.

In final five minutes, add the following on top of rice:

baby carrots   broccoli
cauliflower   green pea pods

Eat plain, or add sweet and sour sauce:

3 Tbsp. lemon juice
1 Tbsp. tamari (like soy sauce)
1 Tbsp. honey
1/2 tsp. onion powder

❖   ❖   ❖

Christmas Salad

Combine and serve on green lettuce leaves:

cauliflower (lightly steamed)
frozen peas
red bell peppers (chopped)

Top with green goddess dressing:

1/2 avocado (mashed)
1/4 C. Nayonaise
3 Tbsp. lemon juice
1 tsp. onion (grated)
1 tsp. Spike

Or use red French dressing:

1/2 C. ketchup   1 Tbsp. lemon juice
1 tsp. Worcestershire sauce   1 tsp. onion (grated)

❖   ❖   ❖

CREATIVE COLESLAW
Thinly slice by hand or with a food processor:

celery	green onions	mushrooms
radishes	red cabbage	white cabbage
yellow, red, and green bell peppers		

Toss with coleslaw dressing:
1/2 C. Nayonaise
1/2 tsp. prepared mustard
1/2 tsp. seasoned salt
1 tsp. celery seed *or* poppy seeds

❖   ❖   ❖

FIESTA SALAD
Slice and toss these ingredients:

black olives	cherry tomatoes
green onions	green peppers
green leaf lettuce	

Serve with avocado dressing:

1/2 avocado (mashed)	1/4 C. salsa

Or use green goddess dressing:

1/2 avocado (mashed)	1/4 C. Nayonaise
3 Tbsp. lemon juice	1 tsp. onion (grated)
1 tsp. Spike	

❖   ❖   ❖

GARDEN SANDWICHES
Grate these ingredients:

black olives	carrots	cucumbers
green onions	green peppers	radishes

Thinly slice:
 avocados   dill pickles
 tomatoes   lettuce (or use sprouts)

Spread Nayonaise inside wholewheat pita pockets and stuff with above ingredients.

Variations:
1. Use wholewheat tortillas instead of pita.
2. Stuff the mixture in a green bell pepper. Lightly steam just until tender, not *mushy*.
3. Place the mixture, using sprouts, in the middle of a large cabbage leaf. Roll up and fasten with a toothpick. Lightly steam.

❖   ❖   ❖

ITALIAN SPAGHETTI SQUASH
Cut spaghetti squash in half and steam. When squash is very tender, scrape out of shell using a fork or spoon. Spoon sauce over individual servings.

Make tomato sauce by heating organic tomato sauce and Italian seasoning. Add these ingredients raw:
 black olives   grated carrots
 green peppers   mushrooms
 onions   sesame seeds

❖   ❖   ❖

LAYERED SALAD
Layer these ingredients in a glass bowl:
 spinach leaves (chopped)   carrots (grated)
 green peas   radishes (sliced)

Optional: Top with wholewheat croutons.

Serve with thousand island dressing:
  1/2 C. Nayonaise
  1/4 C. ketchup
  1/3 C. cucumber (finely grated)
  1 Tbsp. lemon juice

❖   ❖   ❖

MEDITERRANEAN PASTA
Cook and rinse pasta spirals.

Cut up and add to pasta:
  broccoli   cauliflower   green olives
  mushrooms   red peppers   yellow squash

Toss with small amount of Italian dressing:
  1/2 C. extra-virgin olive oil
  3 Tbsp. lemon juice
  1 clove garlic (minced)
  1 tsp. Dijon mustard
  1/2 to 1 tsp. Italian seasoning

Note: If possible, use 100 percent spinach pasta.

❖   ❖   ❖

MEXICAN FINGER FEAST
Cut:
  broccoli   carrots (sticks)
  cauliflower   cucumbers (slices)

Serve with guacamole dip:
  1 avocado (mashed)
  1 tsp. lemon juice
  1 tomato (chopped)
  1 small can black olives (sliced)

1/2 green pepper (diced)
1/4 C. green onions (chopped)
Mexican seasoning to taste

❖   ❖   ❖

OKTOBERFEAST
In wholewheat pita pockets put:
    sauerkraut
    red cabbage (thinly sliced)
    green peppers (chopped)
    poppy seeds

Saute one onion (chopped) until tender. Add 1/2 C. honey sweetened barbecue sauce to onion. Add this sauce to contents in pita pockets.

Note: Serve with lots of napkins!

❖   ❖   ❖

ORIENTAL EXPRESS
Toss:
    carrots (grated)
    green onions (chopped)
    mung bean sprouts
    red cabbage (thinly sliced)
    snow peas (Chinese pea pods)
    water chestnuts (sliced)

Serve with oriental dressing:
    1/2 C. ketchup (low sodium, honey sweetened)
    2 Tbsp. soy sauce (low sodium)
or
    1/2 C. extra-virgin olive oil
    2 Tbsp. tamari (like soy sauce)

❖   ❖   ❖

PICNIC IN THE PARK POTATO SALAD
Chop red potatoes and lightly steam. Rinse with cold water.

Add the following chopped ingredients:
- black olives
- green peppers
- celery
- onions

Toss with:
- 1/2 C. Nayonaise
- 1 Tbsp. Dijon mustard
- 1 tsp. celery seed

❖   ❖   ❖

THE POPE'S FAVORITE
Lightly steam:
- cauliflower
- red bell peppers
- green beans
- wax beans

Toss with a small amount of Italian dressing:
- 1/2 C. extra-virgin olive oil
- 3 Tbsp. lemon juice
- 1 garlic clove (minced)
- 1 tsp. Dijon mustard
- 1/2 to 1 tsp. Italian seasoning

❖   ❖   ❖

POPEYE'S FAVORITE!
Combine:
- cucumbers (diced)
- radishes (sliced)
- red leaf lettuce
- sesame seeds
- spinach leaves

Serve with Three Green salad dressing (Yasmine Marca).
Combine in blender and purée:
    2 C. spinach leaves (tightly packed)
    3/4 C. fresh parsley (packed)
    3 Tbsp. lemon juice (only if foods are raw)
    1/8 C. herb tarragon vinegar
    1 tsp. dried basil
    1/2 tsp. ground cumin
    1 small clove garlic (chopped)
    1/2 C. extra-virgin olive oil

Note: To keep oils from going rancid, add 400 units of vitamin E to a bottle when first opened.

B
Supplies Checklist

This is a list of the things I used in my own detoxification and rebuilding process. This is an example to refer to, not an exact program to implement. Check with your own nutritionist or health professional to form a list that meets your particular needs.

- ❑ Coffee (not instant or decaffeinated)
- ❑ Desiccated Liver (tablets)
- ❑ Enema Kit
- ❑ EPA/DHA (fish oil, capsules)
- ❑ Glutathione
- ❑ Green-Drink (powder)
- ❑ Fiber Cleanse (powder)
- ❑ Juicer (Champion recommended)
- ❑ KYOLIC garlic
- ❑ Liquid Minerals (multi-mineral supplement, including among others zinc, selenium, magnesium, and copper)
- ❑ Melaleuca Oil (also known as Australian Tea Tree Oil)

❑ Pancreatic Enzymes (any form)
❑ Personal Lubricant
❑ Vitamin A (emulsified)
❑ Vitamin C (powder—ascorbic acid, calcium ascorbate, or sodium ascorbate)
❑ Vitamin E (emulsified)
❑ Vitamin B-Complex (tablets)
❑ Water Purifier (or purchased distilled water)
❑ Zinc (any form)

APPENDIX
C
Resource List

The following books were the most help to me in my own war on cancer.

ATTITUDE

Cousins, Norman. *Anatomy of an Illness as Perceived by the Patient.* New York: Bantam Books, 1983.

Siegel, Bernie, M.D. *Love, Medicine, and Miracles.* New York: Harper & Row, 1988.

Simonton, Carl, M.D., Stephanie Matthews-Simonton, and James Creighton. *Getting Well Again.* Los Angeles, CA: J. P. Tarcher, Inc., 1978.

NUTRITION-NUTRITIONAL THERAPY AGAINST CANCER

Airola, Paavo O., Ph.D., N.D. *Cancer: Causes, Prevention and Treatment—The Total Approach* and *How to Get Well.* Phoenix, AZ: Health Plus, 1972 and 1974.

Bieler, Henry G., M.D., and Maxine Block. *Food Is Your Best Medicine.* New York: Ballantine Books, 1987.

Brennan, Richard O., M.D., with Helen K. Hosier. *Coronary? Cancer? God's Answer: Prevent It!* Irvine, CA:

Harvest House Publishers, 1979.

Diamond, Harvey and Marilyn. *Fit for Life* and *Fit for Life II*. New York: Warner Books, 1985 and 1988.

Donsbach, Kurt W., Ph.D., D.Sc., N.D., D.C. *Metabolic Cancer Therapies*. Huntington Beach, CA: The International Institute of Natural Health Sciences, Inc., 1981.

Fischer, William L. *How to Fight Cancer and Win*. Canfield, OH: Fischer Publishing, 1987.

Gerson, Max, M.D. *A Cancer Therapy: Results of Fifty Cases*. Bonita, CA: The Gerson Institute, 1990.

Harper, Harold W., M.D., and Michael L. Culbert. *How You Can Beat the Killer Diseases*. New Rochelle, NY: Arlington House, 1977.

Haught, S. J. *Has Dr. Max Gerson a True Cancer Cure?* Canoga Park, CA: Major Books, 1962.

Holmes, Marjorie. *God and Vitamins*. New York: Avon Books, 1980.

Jensen, Bernard, D.C. *Tissue Cleansing Through Bowel Management*. Escondido, CA: Bernard Jensen, 1981.

Null, Gary. *Gary Null's Complete Guide to Healing Your Body Naturally*. New York: McGraw-Hill, 1988.

Quillin, Patrick, Ph.D., R.D. *Healing Nutrients*. New York: Random House, 1989.

Reuben, David, M.D. *Everything You Always Wanted to Know About Nutrition*. New York: Avon, 1979.

Robbins, John. *Diet for a New America*. Walpole, NH: Stillpoint Publishing, 1987.

Salaman, Maureen, M.Sc. *Nutrition: The Cancer Answer*. Statford, CA: Statford Publishing, 1984.

Simone, Charles B., M.D. *Cancer and Nutrition*. New York: McGraw-Hill, 1983.

Swope, Mary R., Ph.D., with David A. Darbro, M.D. *Green Leaves of Barley*. Phoenix, AZ: Swope Enterprises, Inc., 1987.

Walker, Norman W., D.Sc., Ph.D. *Colon Health*. Prescott,

AZ: Norwalk Press, 1979.

Wigmore, Ann. *Hippocrates Diet and Health Book.* Wayne, NJ: Avery Publishing, Inc., 1984.

OVERCOMER STORIES

Hunsberger, Eydie Mae, with Chris Loeffler. *How I Conquered Cancer Naturally.* Eugene, OR: Harvest House Publishers, 1975.

Smythe, Benjamin Roth. *Killing Cancer: The Jason Winters Story.* Las Vegas, NV: Vinton Publishing, 1980.

Towner, Bettie. *Cancer Holiday.* Seattle, WA: Greenlake Publishers, 1978.

ADDITIONAL RESOURCE

Fink, John M. *Third Opinion: An International Directory to Alternative Therapy Centers for the Treatment and Prevention of Cancer.* Wayne, NJ: Avery Publishing, Inc., 1988.

Notes

CHAPTER ONE—A WAR STORY
1. John A. McDougall, M.D., *McDougall's Medicine: A Challenging Second Opinion* (Piscataway, NJ: New Century, 1985), page 26.

CHAPTER TWO—PRINCIPLE ONE: KNOW YOUR ENEMY
1. "Top Ten," *U.S. News and World Report,* May 20, 1991, page 94.
2. Ernest H. Rosenbaum, M.D., *Can You Prevent Cancer?* (St. Louis, MO: C. V. Mosby, 1983), page 3.
3. Ronald J. Glasser, M.D., *The Body Is the Hero* (New York: Random House, 1976), page 207.
4. Kurt W. Donsbach, Ph.D., D.Sc., N.D., D.C., and Morton Walker, D.P.M., *Metabolic Cancer Therapies* (Huntington Beach, CA: The International Institute of Natural Health Science, 1981), page 35.
5. Rosenbaum, page xii.
6. The editors of Prevention Magazine Health Books, *The Book of Cancer Prevention* (Emmaus, PA: Rodale Press, 1988), page 1.

7. Patrick Quillin, Ph.D., R.D., *Healing Nutrients* (Chicago, IL: Contemporary Books, 1987), page 127.
8. Rosenbaum, page 1.
9. Paavo Airola, Ph.D., N.D., *How to Get Well* (Phoenix, AZ: Health Plus, 1974), page 55.
10. Richard O. Brennan, M.D., with Helen K. Hosier, *Coronary? Cancer? God's Answer: Prevent It!* (Irvine, CA: Harvest House, 1979), page 160.
11. Virginia Livingston-Wheeler, M.D., and Edmond G. Addeo, *The Conquest of Cancer: Vaccines and Diet* (New York: Franklin Watts, 1984), page 102.
12. Max Gerson, M.D., as quoted by S. J. Haught, *Has Dr. Max Gerson a True Cancer Cure?* (Canoga Park, CA: Major Books, 1962), page 130.
13. Harold Manner, Ph.D., as quoted by Maureen Salaman, M.Sc., *Nutrition: The Cancer Answer* (Menlo Park, CA: Statford Publishing, 1983), page 88.
14. Ann Wigmore, *Hippocrates Diet and Health Program* (Wayne, NJ: Avery Publishing, 1984), page 30.
15. Norman W. Walker, D.Sc., Ph.D., *Colon Health: The Key to a Vibrant Life* (Prescott, AZ: Norwalk Press, 1979), page 1.
16. Walker, page 15.
17. Albert Schweitzer, M.D., as quoted by Haught, page 137.
18. Max Gerson, M.D., *A Cancer Therapy: Results of Fifty Cases* (Bonita, CA: The Gerson Institute, 1990), page 16.
19. Quillin, page 122.
20. Stated in "Cancer and Diet, An East West Foundation Publication" (Brookline, MA: East West Foundation, 1980), page 23.
21. Livingston-Wheeler and Addeo, page 44.
22. Harold W. Harper, M.D., and Michael L. Culbert, *How You Can Beat the Killer Diseases* (New Rochelle, NY:

Arlington House, 1977), page 167.
23. Livingston-Wheeler and Addeo, page 46.
24. Livingston-Wheeler and Addeo, page 42.
25. Donsbach and Walker, page 50.
26. Donsbach and Walker, page 50.
27. Gerson, page 143.

CHAPTER THREE—PRINCIPLE TWO: CUT OFF ENEMY
SUPPLY LINES

1. From "Feeding Frenzy," *Newsweek*, May 27, 1991,
page 47.
2. See Charles B. Simone, M.D., *Cancer and Nutrition*
(New York: McGraw-Hill, 1983).
3. "Feeding Frenzy," *Newsweek*, page 48.
4. Simone, page 129.
5. John Robbins, *Diet for a New America* (Walpole, NH:
Stillpoint Publishing, 1987), page 256.
6. Dale and Kathy Martin, *Living Well* (Brentwood,
TN: Wolgemuth and Hyatt, 1988), page 30.
7. Doug Podolsky, "Eat Your Beans," *U.S. News and
World Report*, May 20, 1991, page 70.
8. Paavo Airola, Ph.D., N.D., *How to Get Well* (Phoenix,
AZ: Health Plus, 1974), page 35.
9. Harvey and Marilyn Diamond, *Fit for Life* (New
York: Warner Books, 1985), page 81.
10. Diamond, page 86.
11. Martin, page 26.
12. Norman W. Walker, D.Sc., Ph.D., *Colon Health: The
Key to a Vibrant Life* (Prescott, AZ: Norwalk Press,
1979), page 83.
13. Michael T. Murray, N.D., and Joseph E. Pizzorno,
N.D., *An Encyclopedia of Natural Medicine* (Rocklin,
CA: Prima Publishing), page 78.
14. Ann Wigmore, *The Hippocrates Diet and Health
Program* (Wayne, NJ: Avery Publishing, 1984),
pages 30-31.

15. Murray and Pizzorno, page 78.
16. Wigmore, page 25.
17. Walker, page 4.
18. Bernard Jensen, D.C., *Tissue Cleansing Through Bowel Management* (Escondido, CA: Bernard Jensen, 1981), page 93.
19. Max Gerson, M.D., *A Cancer Therapy: Results of Fifty Cases* (Bonita, CA: The Gerson Institute, 1990), page 190.
20. Linda Rector-Page, N.D., Ph.D., *Healthy Healing* (Sacramento, CA: Spilman Printing Co., 1990), page 32.
21. Wigmore, page 31.
22. Lee Talbert, Ph.D., and Eugene S. Wagner, Ph.D., *Antioxidants: A Powerful Cancer Defense* (American Institute of Health and Nutrition, 1989), page 1.
23. Richard O. Brennan, M.D., with Helen K. Hosier, *Coronary? Cancer? God's Answer: Prevent It!* (Irvine, CA: Harvest House, 1979), pages 139-140.
24. Simone, page 45.
25. Airola, page 222.

CHAPTER FOUR—PRINCIPLE THREE: REBUILD YOUR NATURAL DEFENSE SYSTEM

1. Monsignor José Sebastian Laboa, as quoted in "Panama's Noriega Surrenders to U.S.," *World News Digest*, vol. 50, no. 2563, January 1-5, 1990, page 1.
2. Max Gerson, M.D., *A Cancer Therapy: Results of Fifty Cases* (Bonita, CA: The Gerson Institute, 1990), page 12.
3. Maureen Salaman, M.Sc., *Nutrition: The Cancer Answer* (Menlo Park, CA: Statford Publishing, 1984), page 69.
4. Mary Ruth Swope, Ph.D., and David A. Darbro, M.D., *Green Leaves of Barley* (Phoenix, AZ: Swope Enterprises, 1987), page 112.

5. Ann Wigmore, *Hippocrates Diet and Health Program* (Wayne, NJ: Avery Publishing, 1984), page 18.
6. Swope and Darbro, page 114.
7. Swope and Darbro, page 115.
8. Swope and Darbro, page 122.
9. Norman W. Walker, D.Sc., Ph.D., as quoted by Harvey and Marilyn Diamond, *Fit for Life* (New York: Warner Books, 1985), page 34.
10. Wigmore, page 18.
11. Salaman, page 75.
12. Harvey and Marilyn Diamond, *Fit for Life* (New York: Warner Books, 1985), pages 70-71.
13. Diamond, *Fit for Life*, page 85.
14. Diamond, *Fit for Life II*, page 228.
15. Diamond, *Fit for Life*, page 40.
16. Diamond, *Fit for Life*, page 51.
17. Joel Robbins, D.C., *Health Through Nutrition* (a self-published seminar notebook), page 14.
18. Paavo Airola, Ph.D., N.D., *How to Get Well* (Phoenix, AZ: Health Plus, 1974), page 284.
19. Diamond, *Fit for Life*, page 52.
20. Airola, page 285.
21. Airola, page 285.
22. Robbins, page 15.
23. From "Researchers Trying to Concoct a Tasty Milkshake That Wards Off Cancer," *Colorado Springs Gazette Telegraph*, August 20, 1991.
24. O. Carl Simonton, M.D., Stephanie Matthews-Simonton, and James Creighton, *Getting Well Again* (Los Angeles, CA: J. P. Tarcher, 1978), page 99.
25. Simonton, Matthews-Simonton, and Creighton, page 211.

**CHAPTER FIVE—PRINCIPLE FOUR:
BRING IN REINFORCEMENTS**
1. Charles B. Simone, M.D., *Cancer and Nutrition*

(New York: McGraw-Hill, 1983), page 64.
2. Joel Robbins, D.C., *Health Through Nutrition* (a self-published seminar notebook), page 47.
3. Linda G. Rector-Page, N.D., Ph.D., *Healthy Healing* (Sacramento, CA: Spilman Printing Co., 1990), page 13.
4. Max Gerson, M.D., *A Cancer Therapy: Results of Fifty Cases* (Bonita, CA: The Gerson Institute, 1990), page 215.
5. Michael B. Sporn, M.D., as quoted by the editors of *Prevention Magazine* in "Understanding Vitamins and Minerals" (Emmaus, PA: Rodale Press, 1984), page 34.
6. William L. Fischer, *How to Fight Cancer and Win* (Canfield, OH: Fischer Publishing, 1987), page 191.
7. Patrick Quillin, Ph.D., R.D., *Healing Nutrients* (Chicago, IL: Contemporary Books, 1987), pages 138-139.
8. Linus Pauling, Ph.D., as quoted by Lee Talbert, Ph.D., and Eugene S. Wagner, Ph.D., *Antioxidants: A Powerful Cancer Defense* (n.p.: American Institute of Health and Nutrition, 1989), page 20.
9. Jonathan V. Wright, M.D., *Dr. Wright's Book of Nutritional Therapy* (Emmaus, PA: Rodale Press, 1979), page 302.
10. Shigetoh Miyachi, Ph.D., speaking at the Thirty-Fifth Chlorella Science Symposium, 1983.
11. Jane Brody, *New York Times*, September 4, 1990.
12. Willem H. Khoe, M.D., Ph.D., *The Khoe Newsletter* (special issue).
13. Rector-Page, page 17.
14. Marjorie Holmes, *God and Vitamins* (New York: Avon, 1980), page 282.
15. Harold W. Harper, M.D., and Michael L. Culbert, *How You Can Beat the Killer Diseases* (New Rochelle, NY: Arlington House, 1977), page 46.

CHAPTER SIX—PRINCIPLE FIVE: MAINTAIN MORALE
1. Norman Cousins, *Anatomy of an Illness* (New York: Bantam, 1981), page 45.
2. Ruth Heidrich, as quoted by Beverly Creamer, "A Race for Life," *The Honolulu Advertiser*, March 11, 1991.
3. Bernie S. Siegel, M.D., *Love, Medicine and Miracles* (New York: Harper and Row, 1986), page 25.
4. The British Medical Association, as quoted by Richard O. Brennan, M.D., *Coronary? Cancer? God's Answer: Prevent It!* (Irvine, CA: Harvest House, 1979), page 167.
5. Siegel, page 24.
6. Siegel, page 24.
7. O. Carl Simonton, M.D., Stephanie Matthews-Simonton, and James Creighton, *Getting Well Again* (Los Angeles, CA: J. P. Tarcher, 1978), page 210.
8. Michael McGinnis appearing in "Eat Smart," a MacNeil/ Lehrer special television production.
9. *The Speaker's Sourcebook*, Glenn Van Ekeren, ed. (Englewood Cliffs, NJ: Prentice Hall, 1988), page 212.
10. Cousins, page 85.

CHAPTER SEVEN—PRINCIPLE SIX:
CAREFULLY SELECT YOUR PROFESSIONAL HELP
1. Richard O. Brennan, M.D., with Helen K. Hosier, *Coronary? Cancer? God's Answer: Prevent It!* (Irvine, CA: Harvest House Publications, 1979), page 83.
2. *The Encyclopedia Britannica*, vol. 5 (Chicago, IL: William Benton, Publisher, 1970), page 662.

Health*Quarters* Ministries

HQM functions as an education and resource center for achieving better health through nutrition and related forms of natural health care. Major products and services available directly from HQM include:

◆ Health*Quarterly* A newsletter sent to a worldwide audience. It includes nutrition information, stories of people who have used nutritional therapies to overcome various diseases, thoughts and quotes from various health-care professionals, and personal insights from the Frähms.

◆ Health Resources List A regularly updated document containing the names, addresses, phone numbers, and pertinent practice information for thousands of professionals (M.D.s, D.O.s, N.D.s, nutritionists, chiropractors, colonic therapists, etc.) across the U.S. and Mexico who utilize nutrition and other nontoxic therapies to help people.

◆ The Frähms' other books and tapes *Healthy Habits* (book), *Reclaim Your Health* (book), *The Anne Frähm Story* (cassette).

◆ Anne's Speaking Engagements   A highly sought-after speaker, Anne travels throughout the nation telling her story and lecturing on nutrition and natural health. If you're interested in inviting her to speak in your locality, call for booking information.

◆ Health*Quarters* Ministries Lodge Program   A ten-day residence program at the HQM Lodge, in Colorado Springs, in which participants learn and begin to put into practice specific diet and lifestyle changes aimed at helping them win back their health. (See following page.)

For more information, write or call:

Health*Quarters* Ministries
4141 Sinton Road
Colorado Springs, CO 80907
719-593-8694

Health*Quarters* Lodge

Concept: A place to get away and to focus on learning and beginning to put into practice certain dietary and lifestyle changes that enable the body to move toward improved health

Program:
- ten-day stay (leaving on the eleventh day)
- seven-day juice fast, accompanied by internal cleansing process
- nutrition classes
- product education
- health-food store field trip
- prayer classes
- mild exercise and relaxation
- massage
- "Going Home" dietary plan and menus
- optional "Going Home" supply of key supplements

Important Note: The HQ Lodge program does *not* include doctors, nursing care, drugs, or medications. It is *not* a hospital, clinic, treatment center, or hospice. The staff does *not* label symptoms or illnesses, prescribe drugs, or treat disease. The HQ Lodge *is* an education and lifestyle-change resource center, led by a team of educators and nutritionists. The design of the program fully involves participants in "hands-on" applications of what they're learning, in order for them to make health-promoting changes at home. Health*Quarters* Ministries *is* an organization guided by Christian values and principles, incorporating a Biblical viewpoint into all it does and teaches.

For more information,write or call:

Health*Quarters* Ministries
4141 Sinton Road
Colorado Springs, CO 80907
719-593-8694

About the Authors

David and Anne Frähm have won a platform for helping others battle cancer by successfully fighting that war themselves. Both have since received their credentials as Certified Natural Health Professionals. In addition, Dave has been ordained as a Minister of Health through the Christian Restoration Fellowship International, and has earned N.D. (naturopath) status.

Besides being nationally sought-after educators and lecturers in the fields of nutrition and natural health, Dave and Anne are the founders and directors of the nonprofit organization Health*Quarters* Ministries.